Crazy Visitation

To Sonia,
Peace & good health —
Saundra Murray Nettles
9/20/01

Crazy Visitation

A Chronicle of Illness and Recovery

Saundra Murray Nettles

The University of Georgia Press

Athens & London

Published by the University of Georgia Press

Athens, Georgia 30602

© 2001 by Saundra Murray Nettles

All rights reserved

Designed by Erin Kirk New

Set in 10 on 16 Berkeley Oldstyle Medium

Printed and bound by Maple-Vail

The paper in this book meets the guidelines for
permanence and durability of the Committee on
Production Guidelines for Book Longevity of the
Council on Library Resources.

Printed in the United States of America

05 04 03 02 01 C 5 4 3 2 1

Library of Congress Cataloging-in-Publication Data

Nettles, Saundra Murray.

    Crazy visitation : a chronicle of illness and recovery /
Saundra Murray Nettles.

       p. cm.

    Includes bibliographical references.

    ISBN 0-8203-2299-7 (alk. paper)

    1. Nettles, Saundra Murray—Health. 2. Brain—Cancer—
Patients—United States—Biography. I. Title.

RC280.B7 N465 2001

362.1´969948´0092—dc21

[B]   00-054493

British Library Cataloging-in-Publication Data available

To my daughters, Kali and Alana Murray

To my mother, Edna Lewis Rice

To the memory of my father, George H. Rice Sr.

R.S.V.P.

We couldn't come to our own party.

We were too busy
loving and working,
running on roads
that never crossed.

Perhaps we could have—
should have—
celebrated
just once before

> Time recycled
> the seasons into neat
> bundles, onescore and ten,
> wrapped in gossamer.

Comes now a summons:

Dressed as you are
in the glow of memories
undimmed
by all the years,

Fate requests the honor of your presence.

Contents

✵ Foreword

And men ought to know that from nothing else but thence (from the
brain) come joys, delights, laughter and sports, and sorrows, griefs,
despondency, and lamentations. . . . And by the same organ we become mad
and delirious, and fears and terrors assail us, some by night, and some by
day, and dreams and untimely wanderings, and cares that are not suitable,
and ignorance of present circumstances, desuetude and unskillfulness.
All these things we endure from the brain, when it is not healthy . . .
—Hippocrates, "On the Sacred Disease," ca. 460–377 B.C.

By asking me to write the foreword to this fascinating book,
Professor Saundra Nettles has granted me a great privilege for a second time. The first time was when she asked me to remove the tumor, a meningioma, that was holding her brain and mind hostage.
Over many years this meningioma had grown silently from a single
rogue cell within the arachnoid layer that envelops the brain to a large
mass that laid claim to her left frontal lobe. In January 1995, it un-
equivocally declared its presence with a seizure that left Professor

Nettles unable to speak fluently or to move her right arm or the right side of her face. In the previous months to years, however, the tumor had insinuated its malicious intent on numerous occasions. As Professor Nettles so eloquently describes in this book, prior to the generalized seizure of January 14, 1995, she had suffered numerous unrecognized focal seizures that had taken away her speech temporarily. She had also experienced a subtle but progressive deterioration in her mood, her capacity to perform tasks in an orderly fashion, and her self-awareness. After I removed the meningioma, it took Professor Nettles's brain and mind a long time to repair the damage done by the tumor. But repair it she did, and this beautiful book is the lyrical proof of her magnificent achievement.

It was with more concern than usual that I embarked on Professor Nettles's operation the morning of January 19, 1995. In the archives of the Johns Hopkins Hospital, the operation is described in standard neurosurgical terminology as a "left frontotemporoparietal craniotomy for resection of a left frontal meningioma." The morning of surgery, I would have better characterized the procedure as a "critical attempt to rescue the personality, intellect, speech, and movement of a brilliant academician and wonderful human being." Like my fellow neurosurgeons, I always perform my surgeries determined to protect and preserve every single brain artery, vein, nerve, and precious iota of tissue that I encounter. Although I was certain that with God's help I would be able to remove the meningioma completely, I was determined to do so without disturbing Professor Nettles's precious left frontal lobe. That day God blessed both of us with a successful operation that enabled Professor Nettles to start her long and arduous recovery.

There is much that we know—and also that we still do not know—about the functions that reside in the left frontal lobe, which is the region of the brain most affected by her tumor. The human brain is made up of four major structures: the cerebrum, diencephalon, cerebellum, and brainstem. The cerebrum is divided by a deep cleavage down the middle of the brain into right and left halves called hemispheres. Each cerebral hemisphere in turn is made up of four regions called lobes, namely the frontal, temporal, parietal, and occipital lobes. In most people we identify the left hemisphere as the "dominant hemisphere" because the areas for speech production and for understanding language reside in the left frontal and temporal lobes, respectively.

Although all cerebral lobes have important functions, the frontal lobes are what make us human. The human frontal lobes take up more room by far than any other part of the brain and represent more than one-third of the entire surface of the brain. Although the frontal lobes are relatively small and uncomplicated in lower vertebrates, such as fish and amphibians, they become proportionally bigger and more convoluted in higher primates and in humans. They are responsible for the development of the complex thoughts and emotions that characterize us. Some complex behaviors that may result from frontal lobe damage are: (1) loss of motivation or the inability to form short- and long-term plans, (2) alteration of mood (either depression or inappropriate cheerfulness), (3) apathy or decreased emotional expression, (4) impaired self-awareness, (5) lack of social restraint, and (6) outbursts of irritability.[1]

Over the past two centuries researchers and clinicians have learned much about the complex functions housed in the frontal lobes. Researchers have painstakingly elucidated these functions by either electrically stimulating or removing portions of the frontal lobes in laboratory animals and observing the consequences. Clinicians have confirmed these findings at the bedside in patients with frontal lobe tumors, strokes, or traumatic injuries. We now know that the posterior boundary of the frontal lobe consists of a continuous strip of tissue that controls movement of the opposite side of the face and body. For instance, an injury to this part of the left frontal lobe will paralyze the right side of one's face as well as one's right arm and leg. We call this a hemiparesis if some movement is preserved—as was the case with Professor Nettles—or a hemiplegia if the paralysis is complete. These clinical terms are derived from the Greek prefix *hemi*, meaning "one-half," and the Greek words *páresis* and *plégē*, meaning "a letting go" and "blow," respectively. We also now know that a small island of tissue on the side of the human left frontal lobe controls the ability to speak. An injury to this area will render one unable to articulate fluently. We call this an expressive aphasia, from the Greek prefix *a*, meaning "without," and the Greek word *phánai*, meaning "to speak." It is described as "expressive" to differentiate it from a receptive aphasia, which typically consists of the inability to understand language that results from an injury to the posterior left temporal lobe. Patients with an expressive aphasia, like Professor Nettles, know exactly what they want to say but are unable to say it well or at all. Instead, they utter unintelligible sounds or simply say the wrong thing.

Clinicians have also established that the frontal lobes play a major role in determining complex behaviors and emotions. Some describe the frontal lobes as the seat of one's personality. Recently it has become increasingly apparent that patients with moderate frontal lobe injuries display complex emotions that are most likely a direct result of the frontal lobe injury and not a secondary psychological response to the same. For instance, psychiatrists at Johns Hopkins in the early 1980s found that patients who had suffered a stroke involving the left frontal lobe had a greater incidence of depression than those with strokes in other parts of the brain. By contrast patients with right frontal lobe strokes were more prone to inappropriate cheerfulness.[2] Although these results have been supported by some investigators and questioned by others, they are particularly intriguing in the light of Professor Nettles's story. As the tumor grew and compressed her left frontal lobe, she developed a moderate depression that did not respond to treatment with either medicines or psychotherapy. After the tumor was removed, however, her depression vanished.

Studies such as the one of depression and inappropriate cheerfulness in frontal lobe stroke patients bring us closer to understanding the mind/brain dichotomy, which is still one of our most intriguing but elusive philosophical and scientific concerns. Simply expressed, we know that we have a brain, an organ, and we are aware that, residing in the brain but distinct from it, we have a mind, a sense of oneself as a thinking, feeling being; but we still do not understand how the mind arises from the brain. We still do not know, for instance, how a cluster of nerve cells in the left frontal lobe gives birth to memorable metaphors and poems, such as those in Professor Nettles's book. Although we have made tremendous progress teasing apart and understanding the components and workings of the brain, and we have cultivated in numerous forms the creations of the mind, we still do not know how the one is related to the other.

Seizures played a prominent role in Professor Nettles's story. The brain is an electrical organ because its one trillion nerve cells communicate continuously with one another by generating tiny electrical discharges. The cumulative electrical activity of the nerve cells in the brain is so strong that it can be picked up on the scalp with electrodes, which is what an electroencephalogram or EEG is. The electrical discharges of nerve cells are typically discrete and well organized, but when nerve cells become irritated, they voice their protest by generating increasingly stronger and disorganized electrical discharges. When these discharges reach a threshold, a seizure occurs. Most of us envision a seizure as rendering the individual unconscious and causing him or her to shake all extremities uncontrollably. This is referred to as a "generalized" seizure. Most seizures, however, are more limited and are described as "focal" seizures. When a focal seizure involves the speech area of the left frontal lobe, it literally renders the patient speechless. These focal seizures may last seconds to minutes and are typically very subtle, as in Professor Nettles's case. Her tumor irritated the nerve cells in her speech area and caused her to have numerous episodes of speechlessness. Eventually, however, these irritated nerve cells generated a massive electrical discharge that caused her to have a generalized seizure, lose consciousness, and collapse.

Seizures have fascinated observers since antiquity. To my knowledge, the earliest clinical description of a seizure is found in the ancient Babylonian medical diagnostic series known as *Sakikku* ("All Diseases"), which was compiled between 1067 and 1046 B.C. The

Babylonians and Assyrians called this condition *miqtu* or *miqit šamê*, which means "falling disease of heaven," because they thought that it was the result of possession by a demon or departed spirit.[3] Like the Babylonians, the ancient Greeks concluded that the affected individuals had been temporarily "seized" by a spirit and described them as having "the sacred disease." Indeed, the modern term for recurrent seizures is epilepsy, which is derived from the Greek words *epí* and *lambánein,* meaning "over" and "to seize," respectively. It was Hippocrates, the Greek healer-philosopher born on the island of Cos around 460 B.C., who first proposed that epilepsy was "nowise more divine nor more sacred than other diseases" and declared that "the brain is the cause of this affection."[4] His discussion of this condition in his treatise "On the Sacred Disease" is therefore one of the first modern attempts to address the mind/brain dichotomy.

Insofar as Professor Nettles's book is an intriguing exploration of the mind/brain dichotomy, it is as valuable as Hippocrates' treatise or as the study of patients with frontal lobe strokes that I cited earlier. It creates a portal that allows us to marvel at the mind/brain continuum and may bring us a step closer to resolving the dichotomy. I do not mean to imply, however, that her story is just a neurological case study. When I first met Professor Nettles in the hospital, she immediately impressed me as a strong, determined, honest, and kind individual. I then learned that she was also an accomplished academician and a poet. All these characteristics are evident in her book. It is insightful, honest, and lyrical, and it transcends the simple description of a medical event. It will undoubtedly be of great interest to physicians, nurses, and other medical workers, because we all need to be constantly reminded of the patient's perspective so that we can better serve him or her. But it also will be of interest to readers who want to explore the many issues raised by this narrative, such as the resilience of our spirits and the importance of our family and friends in response to the perplexing vagaries of fate. Above all, this book will be appreciated by all of us who want to be inspired to carry with dignity our common burdens. I for one am tremendously indebted to Professor Nettles for allowing me to be her neurosurgeon, for granting me the honor of writing this foreword, and for sharing with me and her readers her inspirational story of suffering and ultimate achievement.

Rafael J. Tamargo, M.D., F.A.C.S.

Notes

The Greek etiologies of medical terms are derived from *The Random House Dictionary of the English Language,* 2d ed.

1. D. T. Stuss, C. A. Gow, and C. R. Hetherington, "'No Longer Gage': Frontal Lobe Dysfunction and Emotional Changes," *Journal of Consulting and Clinical Psychology* 60 (1992): 349–59.

2. R. G. Robinson, K. L. Kubos, L. B. Starr, K. Rao, and T. R. Price, "Mood Disorders in Stroke Patients: Importance of Location of Lesion," *Brain* 107 (1984): 81–93.

3. J. V. Kinnier Wilson and E. H. Reynolds, "Translation and Analysis of a Cuneiform Text Forming Part of a Babylonian Treatise on Epilepsy," *Medical History* 34 (1990): 185–98.

4. Hippocrates, "On the Sacred Disease," in *The Genuine Works of Hippocrates: Translated from the Greek with a Preliminary Discourse and Annotations,* ed. F. Adams, vol. 2 (New York: William Wood & Company, 1886), 325–46.

❆ Crazy Visitation

Prologue

They seem not to break; though once they are bowed /
so low for so long, they never right themselves.
—Robert Frost, "Birches"

Nearly four years to the day since surgeons removed a large tumor from my brain, I am in my study looking out at the damage from yesterday's ice storm. In my front yard are two birches, one on either side of the stairs to the sidewalk, and they are coated limb by limb with an inch of ice. The weight of the ice causes them to rest delicately on my neighbor Marcia's car. "Birches are made to bend," she said when I called to tell her the trees might damage her car. "Perhaps both your trees will return to their original state." One of them did; I will have to remove the other because the trunk tore at a forty-five degree angle, splitting nearly in two in the process.

Like the birch that righted itself, I recovered from the tumor that grew up with me, undetected by doctors I consulted over many years, pressing into areas of my brain that affected my thinking, speech, and emotions. As an African American woman, I was no stranger to the stress occasioned by gender and race, and early in my career as a scholar had written extensively about the twin evils of racism and sexism. But I was totally unprepared to deal with yet another threat. Unlike diabetes, hypertension, breast cancer, and lupus—diseases that exact a toll on black Americans out of proportion to their presence in the U.S. population—brain tumors are indifferent to social categories.

As I looked at the birches, I asked myself why did I bend and return whole, while others under equally harrowing conditions break in spirit, becoming bitter, angry, or depressed? Was my good outcome simply due to the passage of time, aided by favorable life circumstances at the outset? Was it caused by something I did that others can replicate? Was I the beneficiary of the support and skill of others, or did my recovery come from the grace of God?

One of the ironies of my story is that I had always asked these questions of other people's lives. As a researcher, I was investigating the concept of psychological resilience while the tumor was scrambling my central nervous system. When I was able once again to think abstractly after the tumor was removed, the questions remained, only now I was both participant and observer.

Resilience has a multitude of meanings.[1] Biological resilience is the body's capacity to bounce back from illness. Investigators are identifying various processes, called "protective mechanisms," which work spontaneously or with intervention to offset the effects of assaults to physical well-being. But research has not answered definitely the question of how the brain recovers. Studies support a handful of models that may have a common, as yet unknown, link. One is that with time, deficits following injury can return to normal, provided that the injury is not of a severe type. Still another is that unused parts of the brain do the work of damaged parts.

Fortunately, the brain has its own mechanisms of resilience. In this book, I describe what I did to make sure I did not get in the way of my brain's capacity for recovery.

✄

Psychological resilience is a process that results in an individual's successful mental and social functioning despite adversity. This meaning of resilience comes from studies of people who function well in the face of multiple stresses, such as those that accompany poverty, or who emerge from traumatic experiences and return to former levels of competence. Researchers identify three phenomena in this meaning of resilience: successful social and cognitive development in the presence of threats (such as low birth weight or poverty) to normal progress; effective coping despite adversity; and recovery from traumas, like physical violation and captivity, which overwhelm the individual's ordinary ways of adapting to life's changes. Recovery occurs when symptoms of trauma abate, typically with the aid of supportive caregiving.

Studies that follow people over time have identified several characteristics of resilient individuals, including a strong sense of being able to control one's own fate (known as "personal control" or "internal locus of control"), good problem-solving skills, and effective social skills that enable the person to develop networks of family and friends. Many of these resources are ones that most people acquire in the normal course of development. This observation is the basis for self-help books that offer suggestions on how to develop resiliency, a condition or trait believed to render a person relatively invulnerable, or resistant, to stress.

But the how-to books rarely mention that psychological resilience depends in some measure on a healthy brain. Although feelings of sadness and despair are expected following such events as the death of a loved one, chronic depression can put a person at risk for a host of maladaptive outcomes. When a person has a brain tumor, access to many of the skills tapped by IQ tests, such as the ability to judge and to compare, is often disrupted.

In this book I examine resilience through the lens of the illness that threatened me at mid-life. Because some of my symptoms were lapses in memory and altered personality, I reconstructed my personal history from many sources: my journals; to-do lists and calendars; my recollections and those of witnesses; correspondence; creative writings; and medical records. This book, then, is as much about gaps that the tumor created in my narrative as it is about the events and experiences that I remember.

I do not reduce resilience to a list or a formula. For me, resilience was a continuous set of transactions between conditions that harm and conditions that protect, played out in a real life filled with the stresses of being alive: separation from ones you love or used to love; illness; job change or loss; and all manner of declines. The poet Mary Oliver reminds us that "No one gets out of it, having to / swim through the fires to stay in this world."

One last meaning, which I would discover through my own experience, was resilience as transformation, the capacity for the individual to emerge renewed, sometimes stronger, after calamity. As one of my friends told me, "Suffering refines you." I began reading stories written by people who had encounters with catastrophic illness or the stress of normal turning points in life. At the same time, I started to piece together the events and circumstances of the illness that led to the traumatic moment of finding out I had a brain tumor. My transformation began when I grieved for obvious losses of health and income, and for other losses that were more subtle, such as the sense that I was on-time in my accomplishments and keeping apace with my peers, the feeling of invulnerability, and the certainty of infinite time.

I longed for a veteran voice as I sorted through the symptoms and aftermath of the tumor, but firsthand accounts are rare. I offer my story to those who want a glimpse into the vulnerability created by an unhealthy brain and the restoration of wholeness in the site of secrets and dreams, memory and inhibition, and the origin and ending of all the senses.

✣ You Are Different Now

I open my mouth, but can't form words right now. That's why I'm here: my neurosurgeon, Dr. Tamargo, has prescribed speech therapy. I blink to remove my tears, and rub my left arm; it aches whenever I become anxious. I flush with shame and embarrassment. I wonder if I did so poorly because of the medication. This can't be true.

I listen as the neuropsychologist reviews the results of tests I'd taken a few days earlier. He says that I had trouble with memory, attention, concentration, and fluency in producing words.

The treatment plan gives the facts in terse phrases: "Wechsler Memory Scale-R: Mental control 4/6 *unable to state letters of alphabet. Difficulty counting backwards & counting by threes.* Word Fluency Measures: *10th percentile, mild.* WAIS-E: Digit span, *66th percentile. Avg.*"

I am familiar with the WAIS—the Wechsler Adult Intelligence Scale. I'd administered the instrument, a measure of IQ, years ago when I worked on my doctorate in psychology.

A speech therapist is present for my consultation. She explains how therapy can help me. I will learn some compensatory strategies. My ability to concentrate will be strengthened by various exercises. My ability to retrieve words will improve. They will make videotapes of me as I practice lecturing and give me feedback.

"This is so different from the way I used to be," I say.

"But you are different now," I heard the neuropsychologist say.

"Brain damage?" I ask myself. At the same time, I politely decline his offer of therapy to help me deal with what those scores represent. We talk about my insurance and the number of speech therapy sessions I will need and make plans for physical therapy to alleviate headaches and problems with my jaw.

I walk out of the rehabilitation center with as much dignity as I can muster. Outside, I am barely aware of the sweet scent of May wind. I drive the short distance from the rehabilitation center to my home, walk inside, and call a friend. She had a stroke two or three years before while still in her thirties; she spent months regaining everyday functions. I tell her about my tests and what the psychologist said.

"Saundra," she says gently. "You *are* different now. But different doesn't have to mean worse. Look at me." She had recovered and was back at work. She talks a little about her ordeal and encourages me to be patient and work hard with the speech therapist. When I hang up the phone, I feel more hopeful, but still ask myself, "How did I get here?" I'd asked this question before: I already know the answer.

Five months earlier, on January 14, 1995, I'd become one of one hundred thousand Americans diagnosed that year with a brain tumor.

After seven straight days of driving back and forth on I-95 and the feeder highways that encircle Baltimore and Washington, I was tired. I had given an examination the previous weekend and on Sunday had attended a meeting at the National Science Foundation. Classes would begin the following week. I'd spent three weekdays in my office preparing notes for the courses I taught at the University of Maryland (UM). Finally, I'd completed revisions on a proposal for a new educational research center at Johns Hopkins University, where I had worked on the research faculty for six years before taking the tenured associate professorship at UM six months before.

It was around noon on a cold and sunny Saturday, and I had just returned from the market with food for my daughter Kali, who was home for the weekend. She kissed me hello as I came in the door laden with bags of fresh produce, roasted chicken, and lemonade, and had promptly gone to bed. I planned to take a nap myself.

The phone rang just as I unzipped my jeans. "When did you get back?" I asked as I wriggled out of them. I sat on the bed while Carolyn, a friend, told me about her recent trip to Germany. She had been a research associate at Hopkins, and for three years we had worked with another colleague, Gary, on the evaluation of a multicultural program at a middle school in Pittsburgh. We'd made a good team. Gary was the expert developer of ways to measure personality and attitudes. Carolyn was meticulous; she could spot mistakes in our statistical analyses and endless drafts of reports. I liked to brainstorm, to make connections between phenomena. When I was discouraged about one thing or another, she'd say, "You've done the hard stuff. The rest is details."

I slipped my sweater over my head as Carolyn and I chatted. It was my turn to reply, but when I opened my mouth, nothing came out. I continued to move my mouth, but I could not find words. I felt something in my head spiral upward as if on a very short corkscrew, and I felt myself falling. Later I would learn that I'd had a seizure, that Carolyn had become alarmed as she heard me breathing through the mouthpiece, that she'd called 911, and that she had called Barbara, a close friend who lived near my house in Columbia, Maryland.

The loud knocks must have roused me. I stumbled down the stairs toward the sound. I opened the door. A man in a uniform said, "Ma'am, are you Saundra Nettles?" I stared, opened my mouth, tried to speak. Nothing. I nodded because I recognized the name. The rest comes from a store of sensory impressions received from the barest edge of awareness: the room is filled with many men in uniforms. I sit on a sofa in a room that is familiar, yet I see it through eyes that don't seem to belong to me. "Is this your house?" someone asks. Kali stumbles down the stairs. "What's wrong, Mom? Is something wrong with my mom?" My friend and her dad enter the house. "I'm Barbara Wasik, Saundra's friend."

More questions. I open my mouth, but still cannot speak. The men ask, "Is your mother on drugs? Does she drink?" Barbara and Kali help me put on my jeans. The room is very pretty, filled with pale colors. I am in a garden with roses and green leaves. I stare at the sky. I am on my back, and the sky is blue. The doors shut and I am in a little room that starts to move. The men in uniforms say they want to take me to the hospital.

Eight hours later (although I think it is only a few minutes), the physician in the emergency room says I have a huge brain tumor. The date is January 14, 1995, eight days after my forty-eighth birthday. The preceding months had been full of turmoil—a change from married woman to twice-divorced, single parent; a change of jobs; a change of residence; and the beginnings of the change of life called menopause.

To verify her diagnosis, the doctor holds a negative in front of my eyes. I see images: a dark balloon that is partially hidden by another balloon. "The tumor needs to come out immediately," she says. I have a momentary and massive sense of dread, then nothing. No thoughts. No sweat. No tears. I just sit there, waiting. She continues. "You'll need to go to a teaching hospital. You have a choice of Hopkins or Mary- land." She waited. Six years on the research faculty at Hopkins had given me an insider's view of the making of the institution's reputa- tion; my response was automatic. "Hopkins." It is the last word I re- member saying, although Kali later reported that I'd calmly told her I had a brain tumor and asked her to get rid of the book she had with her, Terry Pratchett's satire *Reaper Man*. Its cover showed a skeleton dressed in red, riding a gray horse and brandishing a scythe. "It freaks me out," I had said to Kali, who told me later that she took the diag- nosis in stride. "I didn't know anything about brain tumors, and I was relieved to find out that there was a real cause. Face it, Mom, you'd been pretty crazy for months."

Barbara was also in the emergency room cubicle. I'd known her for nearly seven years; we'd begun work at Hopkins around the same time and had much in common. When we first arrived, we occupied offices with distinct disadvantages (hers, a former closet, and mine, a dim space adjacent to the copy machine, computer terminal, and bathrooms). We both loved houses and interior decorating and had spent many hours searching for affordable decorative objects. Both of us are short, about five feet. We and our spouses had doctorates in psychology. I don't recall Barbara's presence in the cubicle; Kali said she'd spoken little, as if she were in shock.

I started to cry when a woman in the cubicle next to mine had what seemed to be a heart attack. Kali stepped over and stroked my right arm. "It'll be OK, Mom." Before they wheeled me to the ambulance for Hopkins, I heard the doctor say to Kali and Barbara, "I'd like to know how she's doing."

That day, the symptoms I experienced and the signs the doctors saw coincided in a diagnosis.

※

The beginning of the story of my diseased brain is arbitrary. Literature from the American Brain Tumor Association says that brain tumors can start in the brain or can form from cancerous cells originating in other parts of the body. Tumors, whose growth is abnormal and uncontrollable, can be benign or malignant. Particular types of tumors are defined by grade (the tendency to spread) or a general name that indicates where the tumor arises (adenomas, for example, originate in a gland).

Later I learned that my tumor probably began to grow in late adolescence or early adulthood. With hindsight, I can recognize or interpret certain signs of the diseased brain, and I'll talk about them in their turn. But, nothing I've read, seen, or heard pinpoints the exact time when a person's experience of the world begins to change from normal to nightmare. So I'll begin five months before the diagnosis, near Atlanta, Georgia, where my family had gathered to celebrate its shared roots.

I had looked forward to the party for months, but when I arrived I felt that someone, or something, had taken my place.

※

The booklet compiled for the occasion of the Weems Family Reunion gave the facts: the program's cover bears the date, August 6, 1994, and depicts a tree with the names Alex and Carrie at the roots, and in the branches, the names of their fourteen children. Inside, photographs show our earliest known ancestors—Alex in one, Carrie in the other. Months after the reunion, my father would tell me a little story that the Weems elders recalled. Carrie, bound by law in slavery, was physically bound as well. She was caged; when she was a child someone (her owner? her family?) believed she was wild.

But in the photographs, Carrie and Alex are picking cotton in a field, unshaded except for a single tree. He is old; the sideburns that show beneath the brim of his hat are white, as is the beard that grows in a triangle. A ragged bag is slung over his left shoulder. She stands beside a large basket, already nearly filled with cotton bolls. A jacket is draped across her shoulders; she wears a knit cap. She is staring at something out of the camera's range. Perhaps she is daydreaming.

Alex and Carrie were my great-great-grandparents on my father's side. He was a Cherokee, born a slave in 1854. She, of African descent, was born a slave in 1857. After the Civil War, Alex and Carrie married in 1870 and settled in McDonough, Georgia. A year later, when Carrie was fourteen, they had their first son, Ellie Lee. Ellie Lee was my great-grandfather, the father of Beulah, my grandmother, and Beulah's brother, Ellie, my great-uncle. The photographs of Carrie and Alex that appeared in the reunion booklet were taken by Ellie, and it was he who introduced my parents when my mother came to sit for a portrait in his photography studio in Jacksonville, Florida. My father, who was apprenticing in the Weems studio, was so taken that he followed her to her parents' house and asked their permission to court. They were married in 1944. I was born in 1947.

One hundred and twenty-five years after the marriage of Alex and Carrie, about one hundred of their descendants had gathered at my parents' home near Atlanta. The city's African American newspaper, the *Atlanta Daily World*, described it as the fourth annual reunion and said that most of the family members "live in the surrounding area, but some will come from as far as Ohio, Maryland, New Jersey and North Carolina."

My relatives are working people who, with each succeeding generation, followed the widening path of opportunity for African Americans. Carrie and Alex, who farmed their land, never attended high school. Some of their grandchildren went to normal colleges that were established after the Civil War for the black population and became teachers, served in the armed services, or went north in search of jobs in government offices and factories. My father, Carrie and Alex's great-grandson, attended Morehouse College (as his father before him), and after a try as a full-time photographer, took courses for certification as a mathematics teacher. He taught at Washington High School (Martin Luther King Jr.'s alma mater) until he was promoted to a principal's position. My mother taught kindergarten, and in the 1970s became a reading specialist. They both earned master's degrees in education from Atlanta University.

My cousins and I have a wide range of credentials, from high school diplomas to Ph.D.'s received from schools and colleges either predominantly black or racially integrated. I attended Howard University in Washington, D.C. I graduated in 1967 with honors as a philosophy major, went on to the University of Illinois, where I took my master's in library and information science, and a few years later, returned to Howard for the degree in psychology. One of my cousins sells real estate; another is an elementary school teacher; another is a professor of African American studies. My sister is a professional development specialist for the Atlanta Board of Education, and my brother is an inspector with the health department in DeKalb County, Georgia. The occupations our children now plan to enter are equally diverse—my daughters were preparing for careers in law and education.

The letter recommending my appointment at UM describes me as "a writer, a thinker, and a teacher." I produce lectures, scholarly essays, research articles, poems, and for the last decade or so, chapters for the novel I've been writing. At the time of the reunion, I had two paid positions. One was a nine-month appointment as associate professor of human development at the University of Maryland. The other was a yearly summer appointment as principal research scientist at the Johns Hopkins University Center for Social Organization of Schools.

The living Weems all depend on their intellect, but a strong urge for artistic and mechanical work runs through the family. My father built our house—not in the sense of picking out a builder's model and visiting the site while workers erected preassembled parts but with his hands. From my architect uncle's plans, my father went to the property for months and years, and with helpers, dug the basement, laid the footings, nailed the joists, layered bricks and mortar, cut the drywall. My maternal grandmother earned a private school education for three daughters, with her seamstress skills. My mother sews. At Howard, my evening gowns were the envy of my friends, but my mother's crocheted afghans are prized by all. My daughters collect them from my stash and pile and drape their beds with the colorful zigzags and squares. My house is decorated with other treasures, too. From my maternal grandmother, a crocheted bedspread; from my paternal grandmother, a quilt of squares made from dresses I wore as a little girl; from my great-uncle, a restored photograph of a nineteenth-century black family; from my sister, an abstract acrylic she painted.

Does a propensity to develop brain tumors run in families the way that educational and creative accomplishments (along with brown eyes, long and luxuriously coarse hair, and full lips) run in the Weems? Had I known that my tumor was of a type associated with a chromosomal abnormality[1]—had I known about my tumor at all— I might have looked at my relatives more carefully that day at our reunion and perhaps wondered, did one of my family pass this on to me? Had I introduced a mutation that would affect my descendants? Or was the tumor just a random event, a slub on an otherwise orderly weave: unique, never to be repeated?

My father's sister, Vesta, was the only relative who had been diagnosed with an illness associated with the brain. One Halloween, a blood vessel weakened and tore, and she collapsed at a fair to which she had taken her four children. Two weeks later, she died at age thirty-nine. I was twelve at the time. We lived in the home that is the place of my earliest memories: an apartment that my grandfather, uncle, and father built as a second story over my grandparents' bungalow in Atlanta, on DeSoto Street. When my grandmother called and said Aunt Vesta's condition was worsening, my mother fetched my father, who was working at the site of our uncompleted house. There was no telephone in the one-room shed in which he slept on weekends surrounded by the tools he used to construct the house.

She lived for another two weeks. As a child, I was unaware of the medical procedures used on her behalf. Refined treatment of vascular problems awaited the sixties when the operative microscope was introduced, allowing neurosurgeons close-up views of the nervous system. When Aunt Vesta died, less than a century had passed since the first successful operation on the brain was performed in 1879.[2]

Lying awake in bed, I sensed my aunt's passing. During my early childhood she had not yet had children, so I enjoyed her company when she came to visit my grandparents. The wife of a mathematics professor at Albany State College in Georgia, she taught elementary school after she graduated from Spelman College. We shared a love of books and music. I danced and sang while she played on her ebony grand piano, which was, along with the sofa, my grandfather's green vinyl recliner, and a television, the only furniture in the large living room.

My sister, Pat, and I visited her for two weeks the summer before her death, and I had tried to keep my cousins and sister, all younger than I, from being messy and loud as we played in the house and yard all day. Aunt Vesta would pull me aside and say gently, "Take it easy, Saundra. They're just children." With six active children in her five-room house (my uncle was away during that summer at Ohio State, working on his Ph.D.), she was exhausted at the end of each day and would fall asleep in the bathtub filled with water. I used to try to awaken her; I wanted to keep her from drowning.

For decades after she died, I felt guilty and feared that I too would have a brain aneurysm. At the same time, I sought to atone, evoking her memory while I worked to accomplish good grades or a nuanced performance on the piano. I found this entry, dated April 9, 1983, in my diary:

> All these years have I paid her back because she gave me books
> and attention and did I contribute to her death? I have often
> thought, perhaps because of this, that I would die at thirty-nine
> or at least young, before my children grew up. That I have to pay
> because I saw how tired she was all the time.

Once I turned forty, I stopped thinking I would die without warning.

At the Weems reunion, I can remember that I greeted two of Vesta's children with smiles and hugs. Smiles and hugs, and the occasional "Hi, glad to meet you!" were all I seemed able to do or say that day. I can remember the proceedings clearly enough: the prayer, my second cousins—the youngest generation—singing and rapping on the back porch that served as a stage, the quiz about relatives who were locally renowned, and my father's prayer and remarks before we ate a catered feast of chicken, ribs, and all the trimmings. One of my cousins brought large albums filled with photographs of her children and other relatives. Alana and Kali, my twin daughters (the first twins among the Weems), did not come to Atlanta with me; they were busy with things that active nineteen-year-olds do. It hadn't occurred to me to bring recent photos of them; but I ran into my parents' house, took two from the wall, and passed them around to compliments about how pretty my girls were.

I took some snapshots with one of those cameras you use once and discard after the prints are processed. I didn't know when I would see my relatives who weren't in my immediate family. The three preceding reunions had drawn relatives who lived in Atlanta and its environs; I hadn't attended those. Aside from reunions, relatives in my father's and grandmother's generations kept in contact from time to time, and through them succeeding generations connected. Since the death of my grandmother, Ellie Weems's sister, my cousins, aunts, and uncles had rarely been together at the same time. While she was alive, three generations lived in the Atlanta house she owned with my grandfather. Her home was a gathering place for Sunday dinners of fried chicken, rice and gravy, candied yams, and yeast rolls. I knew in an emergency I could count on the prayers and goodwill of my extended family, but none of us had accumulated wealth beyond the payoff of decency and hard work. I'd never expected nor received much in the way of money or things from relatives other than my parents.

I can't recall much of the narrative in my mind that day at the reunion—I seemed to have little awareness of the internal conversations we call thought. As I sat in the warmth of the sunlight and the family and friends gathered, I glanced at the program with the tree on its cover. Inside, one page was labeled "In Memory Of. . . ." One of the departed was Troy Weems, the last child born to Carrie and Alex. He lived ninety-four years—from 1892 until 1986. At the reunion, I had been introduced to hardy people who I knew must be in their seventies and eighties. From the printout of the family tree stored in my father's computer, I knew that longevity runs in the Weems family. The descendants of Carrie and Alex seldom died young. Carrie herself was ninety-seven when she died. In old age she was bent and stooped with osteoporosis; we could see eye-to-eye. I, too, now expected to live long, age with grace and dignity, and rock my grandbabies to sleep.

※

A day or so after the reunion, my mother drove me to the airport for my return to Baltimore, and we chatted until boarding time. We kissed each other goodbye. As I walked down the skyway to the plane, I pretended I was tethered to a string that allowed me to move without losing balance or appearing to be drunk. That pretense was a habit; earlier in the year, I'd noticed that my equilibrium was slightly off. My head felt as if it were lined with cotton candy, which shifted slightly whenever I moved. I willed my hands to grip my bags, a briefcase in the right one and an overnight bag in the left; my hands seemed to be losing strength and I feared that I would drop something. In college I was diagnosed as having bursitis, and I thought that this disorder (or perhaps arthritis, which runs in the family) had begun to make more than an occasional appearance. I was relieved when I reached my seat.

Perhaps at that point I reflected that every aspect of the person I recognized as myself was changing. Sometimes the changes stunned me and I would ask myself, "What's happening here?" More often than not, I felt unwell and could not communicate the physical sensations and emotions that seemed to dance through me with rhythms of their own.

In the months before the reunion, I'd had a handful of episodes in which my mind was devoid of words. Five months before, in February, I couldn't formulate an answer to a question asked of me in a job interview. On Friday, May 6, a few days before my divorce, I was having trouble finding and speaking words, and at the insistence of my therapist (who thought I'd had a stroke), my daughters had taken me to an emergency room. As I remember, the physician had sedated me, done an EKG, asked if I'd had a history of psychiatric care (I had), said I'd had an anxiety attack, and had given me some Valium and a referral form with an internist's name on it. I don't recall what I said to my daughters when I came out of the emergency room, but they said they weren't informed about any special care I needed; I told them about the Valium.

Over the weekend, I took the medication, slept, and misplaced the referral form. On Monday, I went to my office at Hopkins. I was very lethargic and had difficulty speaking. Four of my friends—among them Carolyn and Barbara—followed me to my office to see if they could help. They knew from my daughters that I'd already been to the emergency room.

The phone rang. My lawyer's voice said, "Saundra?" I opened my mouth, but I couldn't utter complete sentences. One of the women grabbed the phone and spoke: "Saundra's a little anxious. This is her friend Nancy. What do you want to tell her?"

The call concerned my divorce, which would be final the next day.

The lawyers had come to terms and mine wanted to communicate the details. Nancy wrote the messages on a piece of paper, repeated them to me, and I nodded yes or no in reply. At the time, I didn't understand what was happening.

Nancy asked me about witnesses. What witnesses? I was puzzled. Apparently, I'd forgotten that I needed someone to testify about the separation. My friends conferred with each other, checked their calendars, called another friend. Finally, we got witnesses. At the court appearance the following day, I managed perfunctory replies (yes, no, the number of months of separation) and over the course of that week, I recovered my normal cadence of speech—slow, soft, Southern.

Aphasia is the word for my difficulties producing language, although the term is also used for impaired understanding when, say, a person understands words in a strictly literal way and cannot grasp figures of speech. That day in the emergency room, throughout the weekend, and in my office on Monday, I had no trouble following what people said, their nuances of phrase and tone. I could read. I could even move my mouth and vocalize words. But I had large gaps in my sentences. Every part of me knew what I wanted to say. Take water, for instance. I could see a glass of it, hear the sound of it running from the faucet into a bathtub, smell the off-odor of opaque crystals that form in ice trays left in the freezer for too long, feel the tingly bubbles in Perrier on my tongue. But I could not go to the place in my brain that contained the word *water*.

Anomia is the term for the type of aphasia that renders you helpless to find words. There are other types; my inability to speak smoothly was a sign of the deficit called "low verbal fluency." Scientists have studied the various kinds of aphasia for a century and have traced these disorders to specific areas of the brain. Apparently, our knowledge of how the language systems misfire is not complete.

In the months that followed the weekend aphasic episode, I felt sluggish, depressed, and fatigued, but I attributed these sensations to the move my daughters and I made to the house I purchased in June 1994, a townhouse at the end of a row. The development of forty-odd houses is in a forest and is five minutes from a park with a pond called Wilde Lake. Before we moved, Alana, Kali, and I lived for two years in a townhouse I rented. We'd moved there in July 1992 after I left the house I'd shared with my husband. The first year we rented was tough. Kali was a freshman at Hopkins. She'd left high school after the eleventh grade, so she was a year ahead of Alana. She came home on weekends, but I still missed her quirky wit and the columns of books that seemed to accumulate everywhere she sat. Alana was a senior in high school and had just learned to drive. Usually she was upbeat and perky, but the twenty-mile drive to school and a new job at K-Mart seemed to sap her energy. My bills began to stack up like a pile of dirty linen: my half of the mortgage, the rent for my townhouse, medical expenses (glasses for the girls, periodontal treatments for me, a mouth guard to eliminate my tendency to grind my teeth while I slept).

All three of us had to adjust: Kali to campus life; Alana to work and the senior year rush of college applications; I to the single life. I'd thought I would be relieved by the separation from my husband. Instead, my days seemed to consist of depression, exhaustion, and work (I moonlighted as a consultant). Alana stayed with Barbara when I had to go out of town on business. I did not even think about social life. Alana worried about me and tried to help. One day I came home to find a large homemade poster on the refrigerator. Alana had drawn a track with a set of milestones. At the start was a stick figure, labeled "mom," drawn on a yellow Post-it note. Alana explained that we would talk about what I'd accomplished each day and move the stick figure when I met one of the goals. The "mom" figure was halfway round the track when I had aphasia the weekend before the divorce in May 1994. I removed the poster and packed it for the move to our new house in June. I didn't find it for months; I barely had the energy to unpack from the move, and besides, it was time for me to wrap up my work at Hopkins and prepare for the reunion and my new job.

※

Months later, during my recovery from surgery, a friend would write, "My heart goes out to you in this crazy visitation." I now view the phrase as an apt label for the period from the summer of 1992, when I separated from my husband, to the diagnosis in January 1995. "Affliction," one of many definitions of visitation, comes closest to my sense of disease, but "supernatural spirit" also fits the feeling that something had taken over the space where "I" once roamed at will.

✿ Supernatural Spirit

Two weeks after the reunion, I spent August 15, my last day at Hopkins as a full-time researcher, finishing a report and moving the last of my things to my home office. That day, my colleagues gave me an elegant send-off (meaning the usual paper and plastic was replaced with glass champagne flutes and cloth napkins). As the center director made a little speech wishing me well, I held back tears while trying to rehearse the three or four sentences that I would say in reply. I prayed that I would be able to utter the right words. To my relief, the words came out without so much as a stutter. When one of the researchers quipped, "You're going from flying to crawling," I even laughed, although I didn't get the joke until I was well into recuperation: the Hopkins mascot is the bluejay, the University of Maryland's is a turtle, the terrapin.

My transition, however, turned out to be more than a change in symbols. It marked a time when I was still largely unknown to the people around me, when systems and buildings and procedures ceased to have known outlines and details, and when I had lapses of familiarity with myself as a physical, emotional, and intellectual being.

On August 17, I reported to work at the University of Maryland. I was to teach two courses during the fall semester: an advanced undergraduate course, "Adolescent Development," and a graduate course, "Social Bases of Behavior." Each class was to meet once a week for approximately three hours. In the weeks before classes began, I prepared syllabi and initial lectures, and the office staff introduced me to all of the modern devices and the codes needed to use them. But I couldn't seem to get the numbers right. I couldn't remember my voice mail identification and my new extension; I couldn't remember the two lines of instructions that would activate the printer; I scrambled digits in the code that would get me into the campus computer; each time I transmitted a facsimile or told someone my new address and phone number, I had to consult the departmental roster. The sequence of steps and the associated codes needed to access the university's electronic mail, the computerized library holdings, and the Internet were completely beyond my command.

I fared no better off campus. When I went to the ATM, I would punch the wrong buttons and walk away without needed cash. And supermarkets had installed those computerized devices that accessed your bank account or credit card. For months, I repeated this scene every time I paid for food:

I fiddle with my bankcard. Two tries and I still don't get the black stripe to glide along the invisible, electronic swipe line. The cashier rolls his eyes upwards, shifts his weight from one foot to the other. "Here, let me," he says. His voice has a slight edge. I want to get

cash above the amount of my purchase. Somehow I keep punching
the wrong numbers. "How much do you want, Ma'am?" I turn red,
give an amount. Not saying a word, the cashier punches the correct
figure. I walk away, wondering: Is this the way older people are
treated?

Confronted with devices that I couldn't easily master, I seemed to give the technological demands a lower priority than the demands of preparing for my role as a teacher. I told myself that I would get these things right when I had more time. In the meantime, I compensated. To get messages on my voice mail, I kept the brochure with the appropriate digits in full view next to the telephone; every time I needed to print something from my computer, I asked for assistance.

Although I was incapable of considering my adaptation to compensatory strategies, I had become adept at them. I now recall instances in 1993 and 1994: my crutch through these times was my computer, which I had used for five years. Although part of the time I was out in the schools and community centers collecting data, writing reports and other materials was the biggest part of my job.

In meetings I had trouble following the flow of discussion and was preoccupied with staying alert. I had lots of company; many people set their minds free in these settings. I did best when each person had to respond to similar questions. Before I spoke, I wrote the points I wanted to make—even when they were obvious responses (for example, to the question, What is your position in this institution?). When my turn came, I read from notes like the ones below, which I found clipped to my 1994 calendar:

1. resilience

   protective environments

   participate, opportunities to

   social support
2. multicultural

   structures that work
3. science and math

   urban systemic initiatives.

From these notations I have surmised that each person at the meeting was asked to talk a bit about research interests.

✻

Until August 30, the memory problems were bothersome, but not alarming. They became so the first day I met with graduate students. The classroom was hot and all the seats, about twenty-six of them, were filled. Some of the students looked to be as old as I was, and some, a good three decades younger. There were five or six men, a relatively high number for a course in the College of Education, where women predominate. Asian and African American students were in the minority.

I took a deep breath and gripped the edge of the lectern to steady myself. "I am Saundra Nettles, your instructor for this course." I felt dizzy, began to perspire. Was it fear? Nervousness? I mentioned something about being new to the university and told them my areas of expertise, reviewed the syllabus, asked and answered questions. So far, so good. "Would each of you please introduce yourself to the rest of the class and to me?"

"David . . ." the first student said. I repeated the name, noted his areas of interest on the class roster, tried to picture his face and name in my mind. Nothing. "Karen. . . ." Again, nothing. I glanced around. Could the students tell that something was wrong with me? They must have noticed. This continued—students repeating their names and specialties, and my taking notes, trying to recall something. In the past, after first-day introductions I'd been able to recall the first names of at least half of my students. But on that particular first day, twenty-six times I came up blank.

These accumulating lapses in memory were signs of failures in systems that in the past had served me automatically and so well. My ability to concentrate was deteriorating; when reading in my office my attention would shift in rapid succession to objects on the book-shelves, conversations in the reception area outside my door, pictures on the wall, dirt on the floor, sounds of car radios on the street be-tween the College of Education building and Cole Field House, where the Maryland Terrapins—our basketball team—played on the home court.

I couldn't focus, for instance, on a phone number long enough for my brain to store it. At times, my thoughts still flew, skimming along the electric fields of my brain. At other times, my mind moved for-ward at a slow crawl. The energy I needed to perform mental work was waning.

�֎

On the Saturday before Labor Day, I went to another family gathering, this one of my family of friends. I was fortunate to have many such families—"fictive kin," as anthropologists call them. I was a participant in two writers' groups. One group met in Baltimore, and the other floated between Washington, Columbia, and Arlington, Virginia. There were friends I'd made from the varied places I'd worked over the years: in the early 1970s, the Moorland-Spingarn collection at Howard, the African American Studies Program at Maryland's Baltimore County Campus, and in the late 1970s and early 1980s, the American Institutes for Research (AIR) in Washington. Friends from these years were scattered across four states. Although months, sometimes years, passed without contact, the emotional bonds—forged from tears, laughter, and long conversations over coffee or wine—were strong enough that with one phone call we'd pick up as if only a day had passed.

That Saturday in 1994, eight of my Hopkins friends met at a home near mine. Each of us brought food. My contribution was Silver Queen corn, which is sweet and tender if you don't boil it more than four or five minutes. Some things you can't forget even if you want to. As I sat on the deck drinking virgin piña coladas because alcohol had begun to trouble me, I remembered that three of the women, including Barbara Wasik, had been in my office four months earlier, when I had lost the ability to find and say everyday words. When it happened that day in May, none of us had thought to apply the word *aphasia* to my temporary disability. On this Labor Day, none of us talked of the past at all. We crowded around a big table in our friend Lori's kitchen. Our conversation was about fresh starts: a business, new work, a child's senior year in high school, decorating a house.

After we ate, we decided to walk off the meal. The air was unseasonably crisp and cool, and we needed jackets. I thought I had left mine in the car and was about to get it when a gloomy spirit visited me. Tears welled in my eyes and spilled down my cheeks.

"Lori," I said. We were in the kitchen, stacking the dishes for cleaning later. She turned to me. "I think I'd better go." The tears continued. I wondered if I could walk on steady legs.

"What is it, Saundra? You think you've had too much of us?" Her voice was light, but I sensed her concern.

"No, I'm just a little tired."

I said my good-byes to the group, which was setting out on one of Columbia's wooded pathways, and went to my car. One minute, relaxed and having fun. The next, crying as if I hadn't a friend in the world. In minutes, the tearburst was over. What brought that on, I wondered? In the car, I'd wailed like a wild thing.

�֎

By the end of the first two weeks of classes, I was having problems with long-term memory. This problem surfaced when I was in the midst of one of my earliest lectures on a subject of great interest among scholars of human development. The topic was resilience, the technical term for positive outcomes despite adversity. A colleague, Joe Pleck, and I had published a major review on resilience, and I had written other articles about young people who live through unenviable circumstances—poverty, terrible illness, academic failure in early life—and who cope with them in admirable ways. I felt unusually comfortable with the material.

During the lecture, the students were attentive; they seemed to enjoy hearing about the varied meanings of resilience: beating the odds in life, surviving unspeakable trauma, or coping from day to day amid severe stressors.

"People can bounce back, can cope successfully, but not at all times in all situations," I said. The students listened. A few had pens poised just above lined pages in the spiral notebooks. "That observation has led researchers to identify the characteristics that protect people in times of adversity and risk. Some characteristics are in the person." I gave a list, defining each item and giving examples.

"Other characteristics are in the person's social environment. One is social support." I paused. Neither definition nor example came to mind. I thought maybe I'd remember if I read from the outline; my usual practice was to prepare an outline with major topics and three or four subheadings under the main points. For details, I relied on material stored in my brain, or noted briefly on the outline.

I tried to find the right place, but could not.

A student raised his hand. "Dr. Nettles, what is social support?"

"It's when. . . . there are several kinds, such as instrumental. . . . it means people help you. . . ." I felt warm, as if blushing. I thumbed through my notes. "I can't seem to recall the complete definition right now. I'll have it for you after the break. Let's move on."

In anticipation of further embarrassing lapses of memory, I resorted to copious notes. That strategy uncovered another problem: writing notes in longhand unaccountably tired me so much that my handwriting would grow progressively smaller until it was barely legible. I would pause many times in the course of a lecture—at one point, unable to recall a pertinent fact or an author's name; at yet another, to grope for a word or two and to find none.

Out of class, recording dates and times in my calendar became a hit or miss affair. This was particularly irksome. Like most busy people, updating calendars and to-do lists was as indispensable to well-being as daily rituals of flossing and brushing. One event that I had remembered to record was on September 12. A reception was being given by UM's Office of Multi-Ethnic Student Education. New faculty members would be introduced, and I saw the event as an opportunity to meet other people of color on the campus. In my own department, I was one of two newly hired African Americans on a full-time faculty of twenty-one persons; I was the first African American in the department to earn a tenured position.

The reception was on a Monday. I had no classes that day and decided to work at home. Until time to leave for the reception, I read research articles. I recall no unusual physical sensations. By this point, feelings of lethargy had become virtually daily companions.

I decided to wear a new dress that I had purchased at a shop whose clothing had an ethnic flair. The dress was a new style for me: a chic, brown cotton-knit tube—one size fits all—with long sleeves and an elastic band that could be raised or lowered anywhere from the waist to below the knee. I applied makeup, using blusher, lipstick, and eyeliner to give a glow to my features and to detract from a new one— dark circles under my eyes that would not go away no matter how many vitamins I took and how much sleep I got. At the time, my hair was shoulder-length, worn in a style called a "wrap." To get it, I wound my freshly-shampooed hair around my head and sat under a dryer. When my hair was brushed out, the ends curved toward my face.

I slipped the dress over my head and hiked the waistband to a point just above my hipline. I am short—about five feet—and the hemline fell right above my knees. I thought it was a flattering length for me. I glanced at myself one last time in the bathroom mirror. I was, as my daughters would say, "good to go."

I took a step from my bedroom, my right hand gripping the iron banister down the curve of the stairs. Then something went wrong.

I am holding the railing as my legs buckle. I slip and slide down the stairs. My head. . . .

I'm at the bottom of the stairs. Something in my head is crowding out all but what I can do right now. I rest my head on the stairwall. My new dress, wet with perspiration, clinging. I must wash it. I stand, let my body settle itself, and like a sleepwalker, walk down another set of stairs to the basement, pull off the dress, place it in the washing machine. I go back upstairs. My body is trying to tell me something.

I called a friend at Hopkins and asked her to have someone call me every couple of hours. I explained that I'd had a fainting spell, and from the fall, a possible concussion. I called the Office of Multi-Ethnic Student Education, expressed my regrets, and slept between phone calls from my friends.

Later that week, I recounted the details of my fainting spell to a close friend. "I think I might be approaching menopause," I said to him. "I'm tired all the time. Can't sleep. I get dizzy. My memory goes bad sometimes." He was concerned about my losing consciousness. "Saundra," he said, "fainting isn't a sign of menopause."

I made an appointment with my gynecologist, who had been my

physician for twenty years. He was the first to have heard the two heartbeats in my womb, the first to detect signs of potential problems that needed follow-up from other medical professionals. I have trusted him.

On September 26, I complained to him about the fainting spell, memory loss, and anxiety. He listened as I reviewed my list of recent stressors. When we met in his office after he examined me, he referred me to a primary care physician for follow up on my general health, and wrote prescriptions for lorazepam (Ativan), an antianxiety medication, and hormone replacement therapy (HRT). The doctor advised me to wait before filling the HRT prescriptions, because he wanted to see the lab results for my hormone levels. Depressed levels can indicate the approach of menopause.

A few days later, my test results indicated that my hormone levels were indeed low and that I should begin the HRT. Beyond the test results, I knew my family history—one of heart disease, hypertension, and stroke on both maternal and paternal sides. Nineteen years before, this same family history had led my doctor to order bed rest for the last six months of my pregnancy. Against this backdrop, hormone replacement made sense.

I went to the library to see what I could find on menopause. I took care to be casual, nonchalant as I checked the call numbers for titles. As I glanced around to see if anyone was watching, I smiled. This was the exact approach I used as a preadolescent looking for books on sex at the West Hunter Branch of the Atlanta Public Library. Now, decades later, I felt somewhat surprised that I viewed a normal developmental transition as if it were something forbidden and shameful, a sign of lost fertility. I was already feeling that I had aged rapidly in the space of a year or so. One of my friends had recently asked if and when I would start coloring my hair. Upon hearing me speak about an aching knee that I thought I injured while roller-skating in my basement, another friend commented, "It's probably old Arthur [arthritis] talking."

Another reminder had just arrived in the mail over the summer. It was the *Psychology of Black Women Newsletter,* the publication of a section of Division Thirty-five of the American Psychological Association. The current president of the section had written a piece reflecting on the status of African-American women within the organization. I was mentioned, which brought back happy memories of organizing and conceiving a new vision of the psychology of women. What jolted me was that the writer cited me as a foremother, a distant figure in the past: "The first step is to remember that none of us got here by ourselves. We owe a debt of gratitude to Black Women who took risks to make opportunities for us. Most of those foremothers are unknown to us, but in the Section, we should take time to thank Dr. Saundra Rice Murray (Nettles), Task Force Chair in 1976–1977; Dr. Pamela Trotman Reid, first Chair of the Committee on Black Women's Concerns in 1978–1979; and Dr. Vickie Mays, first President of the Section, 1984–1986; and countless others whose energy and foresight made it possible for us to have a Section today."

The tribute was touching, but I was not quite ready to be a foremother (with all those surnames!). Perhaps the newsletter reminded me of my feminist roots and the models of wise elders among women in my family and in my profession. None of the women

I admired had ever said a word about menopause. I shrugged my shoulders and thought at least I had a diagnosis: menopause and anxiety. I was taking something that could alleviate both. We weren't talking life or death here.

Besides, I was having some good moments—times when I was both lucid and energetic. Earlier in the month, I had attended a conference on student achievement. I saw many old friends and enjoyed the formal presentations and the informal conversations between sessions and at meals. After the conference, which was in northern Virginia, I'd felt well enough to drive the short distance from the hotel to the shop in Alexandria where I'd purchased the brown dress. On the Saturday before my doctor's appointment, my new colleagues at UM gathered for a party. I picked a chair, settled in, and happily chatted and ate Maryland blue crabs cooked in their hard shells. It is impossible to be erudite as you use your fingers and decide what is edible and what is not. There was little pressure to be anything other than sociable, and I remember feeling the beginnings of friendship when I showed Jamie, a Canadian psychologist, how to dissect the crab.

Shortly after the visit to my gynecologist, I made an appointment to see the primary care physician. I gave the fainting episode little thought. It wasn't until much, much later that I thought to compare that blackout with one that had preceded it by twelve years.

※

It is January 1982. I am in my office at the American Institutes for Research (AIR), preparing the draft of the final evaluation report of the Push for Excellence (PUSH/Excel) program, founded and led by the Reverend Jesse Jackson. The words come slowly. I am distracted by the gray clouds outside my window; as forecast, it would surely snow that day. I am distracted by thoughts of what I have to do. As usual, I move in and out of multiple time zones. The children are on one schedule (a pediatrician's visit and daily routines of day care, bedtimes, meals), and my husband and I constantly check to see whose turn it is to pick them up from day care, to cook dinner, to take the laundry to the cleaners. The AIR zone is layered with my four projects: preparation of a schedule for data collection; a trip to Boston; reading a manual about the Army's occupational specialties; the day after the Boston trip, a meeting in Washington with PUSH/Excel and the U.S. Department of Education. When I think of this one, I shake my head and try to get back on task. The draft of the report I am writing will be an item on the agenda.

After lunch, I attend a meeting. Amid discussion on why the PUSH/Excel evaluation's remaining statistician will be reassigned to another project, I begin to feel dizzy and excuse myself. I walk to the ladies room, meeting my research assistant on the way. I say, "Come with me. I feel funny, and I don't know what's going to happen." We enter the bathroom. My head feels as if it is disconnecting from the rest of me, and I am falling.

When I regain consciousness I am puzzled. Why are all these firemen in this little bathroom? Why is our office manager here? Why does everyone look so grim? I struggle to get up, but someone applies gentle pressure on my shoulders. "Just stay here awhile," he says. Another person jokes, "You must be a valuable person. We got a lot of calls for this address."

I'd been feeling anything but valuable. During my five years at AIR, I'd begun to lose my ability to predict or control when I would be "on," alert, focused, articulate, discerning. Getting a good night's sleep, abstaining from alcohol, eating healthy food, and making time for relaxation did not ensure that I would be fit or ready on any given day. Friends tell me of times that I performed effortlessly, with flair and passion, and of other times when I seemed listless, distracted, irritable, or simply not there. They've talked about conversations we've had, but I have no memory of them.

I had thought, as everyone else had said, that the PUSH/Excel evaluation, which lasted from 1978 until 1982, had tested me severely. I was also exhausted by the convergence of many demands. Motherhood was one. My twins were toddlers at the time I took the job; when I worked on weekends, they often played with toys on the floor of my office. Housekeeping, travel across the country, public speaking, and media attention were additional stressors. In a textbook chapter on the psychology of black women, I'd written, "Being all things to all people—at home and on the job—leaves little time for being oneself."

※

The early days of the study had been exhilarating. With Charles Murray (who later wrote *The Bell Curve*) as principal investigator, and other colleagues, I traveled to the cities that would be covered in the evaluation. The first stop was Chicago and dinner at Jackson's house. I barely ate. At the other sites—Kansas City, Chattanooga, Denver—we did the routine things that go with setting up a national study: making arrangements for data collection, giving overviews of the study, getting to know the people we would work with, visiting school sites.

I understood what charisma meant when I witnessed a rally in the New Orleans Superdome. Jackson led the arena, packed with students chanting, "I am somebody." I had wanted the program to work—to report that a black man got kids back on paths once valued above all else in the black community. Paths that led up the mountain toward jobs, respectability, moral authority. Having been raised in the black Baptist church and having attended predominantly black schools in Atlanta, I felt comfortable with Jackson's message and at ease in the schools that signed up for the project. But Jackson detoured from the domestic to the international. In the midst of efforts to get the multi-city study underway in September 1979, I awakened to a front-page picture in the *Washington Post*. I swore. Jackson and Yasir Arafat, the leader of the Palestinian Liberation Organization, were shown in an embrace. I thought, why did this happen, now of all times? I was well aware of what this would mean for the increasingly tenuous relations between blacks and Jews in the U.S., and for PUSH/Excel, which had thus far enjoyed broad support.

Jackson's gesture was condemned widely, and the program came under intense media scrutiny. AIR's evaluation, which had reported that PUSH/Excel was more social movement than educational program, provided the copy. Murray seemed to relish the attention, but I gave interviews only when I could not refer requests to someone else.

In his 1988 book, *Jesse Jackson and the Politics of Charisma: The Rise and Fall of the PUSH/Excel Program,* Ernest House told his version of the story. House, one of the scholars the National Institute of Education had engaged to study the evaluation, gave the research a mixed review, saying that the evaluators' "training in social science had taught them to see certain things other people could not see; it had also taught them *not* to see things that others could see." House portrayed me as a "tragic" figure, caught between my "superiors" at AIR, and the black community and PUSH, who felt I was a traitor. He said I was a "potential heroine put into a position in which no heroic acts were possible." In his view, a neophyte evaluator, as I had been, should not have had the job.

I considered myself to be a trouper. Although I had my share of limelight duties—meetings with Jackson, attending national conferences of PUSH, reading and hearing about my work in publications like the *New York Times* and the *Washington Post*—most of the work was making arrangements, attending meetings, collecting and analyzing data, writing reports, and traveling to Chicago and the six cities that were part of the evaluation. I met with national and local directors, staff, and supporters of the program. Had I been in the program rather than one of its evaluators, I might have formed some lasting friendships. After the work day was over, the PUSH/Excel staff often invited me and other AIR staff to visit them at home or to sample the cuisine at the best soul food restaurant in town. We would chat about our kids, or about our ideas on race or education or social progress. I even eased off the habit of cursing after I'd been around PUSH/Excel staff, who neither smoked nor swore in my presence. They could get frustrated and angry, especially at the evaluation and with me, the messenger they saw most often. But what I remember most is the commitment to the cause and the spirituality of the people, who saw PUSH/Excel as a continuation of the struggle for racial justice. Prayer was routine at meals, at meetings, and as greetings.

Their ministry affected me. I affiliated with a Baptist church in Washington, and for three or four years attended church regularly with my husband and children; during Sunday services, joined the prayer circle at the altar. I often cried as we held hands and listened to the minister ask for God to bless us.

I had few conversations with Jackson. Members of his staff invited me to participate in morning runs with him and his entourage, but I declined: I smoked, did not ever think to pack anything but business clothes, and had never been known to participate voluntarily in any type of sport. My opinions of Jackson were gleaned from his questions, answers, and actions in meetings, conference speeches, and the radio broadcasts of Saturday morning meetings of the Operation PUSH from its Chicago headquarters. Jackson could get to the core of an issue faster than anyone I have known and would "make it plain" in phrases that anyone could understand, whether or not they believed or accepted it. The "I Am Somebody" speech became my favorite distillation of much of the research on what goes into people's ideas about themselves.

But I saw many individuals struggle with Jackson's vision and the demands of work as advocates. I saw four national directors—respected educators all—come and go over the three years of AIR's evaluation. They left for various reasons: burnout from constant travel, policy disagreements, or the desire to get back to their regular jobs. Viewing their experiences and living my own, I learned a basic lesson about causes and the people who champion them: the cause takes precedence over the individual, or as one of my friends puts it, "One monkey won't stop a show." When people in the organization said something like "Politics is politics; don't take it personally," I knew some sort of public challenge to the findings or the methods was forth-coming.

I welcomed tough questions. As an African American woman born in the late forties, I came of age in the sixties when four great struggles converged: the social movements for civil rights and women's liberation, the protest against the Vietnam War, and the sexual revolution. I was a beneficiary of those upheavals, and I'd paid my share of the costs with the stress of being among the first to test, or make new rules on the job, in marriage, and as a mother. Invulnerability is the delusion of the arrogantly strong, and with the life experiences and professional credentials of a thirty-something black Boomer, I believed I was able to withstand just about anything. I considered myself to be just as brainy, just as motivated, just as energetic as Jackson and Murray. I thought that, with extra effort and a little luck, I could make the kind of impact that they seemed destined to make; their views would soon dominate the national dialogue on race and social class. I expected my contribution would be in either the psychology of women or education reform. But, as the evaluation progressed, I felt that my role was as the perpetual understudy—observing the stars, learning their steps, hoping for a chance someday to step into their shoes so that I could dance to my own beat.

After the 1982 blackout and a later, prolonged bout with an upset stomach, I saw two doctors. They found nothing physically wrong with me. One of the doctors suggested that I stop smoking and read *The Road Less Traveled*. Eventually, I did both.

✳

On October 21, 1994, about three weeks after the blackout when I fell down the stairs in my house, I see a primary care physician. As I complete the form for new patients, I feel the recurring weakness in my right hand. Holding the pen and entering even a few lines tires me.

The nurse takes my blood pressure and checks my weight, which is down a few pounds since September. The doctor checks my reflexes and my eyes, listens to my heart through a stethoscope, and thumps my back. I tell him about my fainting spell, my trip to the emergency room when I lost my speech, my memory problems, the probable arthritis in my hands, and my heart palpitations. He asks if I had an MRI or a CAT scan at the emergency room. "I don't know," I reply.

He connects me to an EKG machine, tells me to go to the lab afterward, where someone will draw blood for other tests, and that he will check the records at the emergency room.

It is Friday, and I don't have classes. I go home. I am extremely tired and go to bed. I want to be rested for Saturday errands and a party for my friend Lori, who is getting married and moving to Albuquerque. I sleep straight through the afternoon, awaken in the evening about 8:00 and eat, then go back to sleep. I awaken about 3:00 the next day. My head feels like it's stuffed with cotton candy. I get dressed, intending to go to the grocery store.

On the way to my car, I see my neighbor, Marcia. I open my mouth to speak and, once again, have difficulty getting all the words out. She says, "I don't think you should be going anywhere just yet. Let's walk around the courtyard." She takes my arm, and we begin to walk past the townhouses on our cul de sac. I try to tell Marcia about events in my life, but I am still having difficulty. I begin to cry. I want to stop, but I cannot control my tears. Marcia says soothing words. We are back at my house. I go inside, call my friends to tell them I am exhausted and cannot come to the party. I go back to bed and sleep all night and most of Sunday. By Monday, I feel OK and am ready for work.

A few days later, the doctor calls. He leaves a message on my answering machine saying that the blood tests don't show anything, but that he still has to contact the emergency room for the records of my visit. I erase the message from the tape. Soon I forget about the call.

※

The two blackouts, I can now surmise, were generalized seizures in which activity spread across the neural circuits in both of my brain's hemispheres. The loss of consciousness from a seizure is one sign of a tumor, as are other physical and mental losses I experienced—loss of memory, loss of speech, loss of balance, loss of strength.

In 1994 and all the years before, I was ignorant of the tumor, advancing, invading cell upon cell, pushing between my skull and the left front of my brain. Had I known, I might have understood, at least occasionally, my lack of panic, fear, or even passing concern at my labile emotions and the other symptoms; or the times when I was outside myself, an observant but inept coach, watching Saundra's every action, making corrections when I could; or the feeling that some other person was in my skin, in my head.

✀ Nourished on Nightmare

Many months after the surgery to remove the tumor, I read these lines in a pamphlet, "Brain and Spinal Cord Tumors," published by the National Institute of Neurological Disorders and Stroke:

> Because they strike at the core of the individual's identity, changes in behavior and personality can be the most frightening and devastating symptoms of a brain tumor. These symptoms usually occur when the tumor is located in the brain's cerebral hemispheres, which are responsible, in part, for personality, communication, thinking, behavior, and other vital functions. Examples include problems with speech, language, thinking, and memory, or psychotic episodes and changes in personality.[1]

I reread the passage. Identity and personality. I had no idea until then that tumors could affect who you think you are—could cause you to lose track of yourself. And this was what had happened to me.

Because I could not trust my memory of the tumorous years, I decided that my journals could tell me something. I gathered all the volumes, from the six-by-nine spiral notebooks used years ago, to the hardbound "blank books" that my daughters and friends had given me as gifts. The first volume was dated November 1982, nine months after my first blackout. By 1994 I'd written more than forty volumes of diary entries, poems, and notes for novels, short stories, and essays.

My resume, appointment calendars, bank statements, marriage licenses, divorce papers, voter registration card—all the other documents of my life tell the story of the person who tried to be a good mother and citizen. The journals tell the story of the person, the self, who was dying.

※

The dreamer in me had known something was up. After the blackout in 1982, I'd had a nightmare and recorded it in the journal:

> The woman walked along busy New Hampshire Avenue
> and turned left onto the path along the stream.
> The stream was clear;
> She could see rocks and plants . . . and a child
> Drowning? Let me help!
> No. The child floated face up
> serene, expressionless.
> The woman walked on the calm water
> about to save the child.
> No. She walked on glass.
> The child was trapped under the glass.

Even then, I'd had the notion that the two people in the nightmare were me, but I'd decided that I could understand it better by transforming the dream into fiction. The note that I wrote in my journal in November 1982 said, *"This story will be about self expression and the death of a self."*

Looking back, I see the dream as the beginning of a breakdown triggered perhaps by the tumor and certainly by what was going on in my life. For the first time, I had failed to meet my own expectations. I had attempted to conduct a clean evaluation; instead, Ernest House and a colleague were about to publish a negative critique of the PUSH/Excel study in a major journal. I tried to conform to the AIR routine of long hours and good work; instead, I heard talk of my being "retooled" to work on defense contracts and had been chastised, unfairly I thought, for my handling of a new project in Boston. I would leave AIR in December 1982. I'd chosen to work as an administrator in the United Planning Organization (UPO), Washington's community action agency.

I had not tried to find work in another think tank. I would have liked to return to academe—I had taught for two years at one of UM's campuses before AIR—but I had only one scholarly publication in the five years I was at AIR. It would take me awhile to get back on the professorial track. Besides, I felt very guilty about the distance I had gone from my roots in the black community. I wanted to disown the privilege of criticizing the honest efforts of my own people.

At UPO, I felt out of place. I went from an office overlooking the canal in the well-heeled Georgetown section of the city to the Head Start centers and homeless shelters in Washington's most impoverished neighborhoods. I was the only Ph.D. in the agency. Within a few months, instead of conducting an evaluation, I found myself vigorously obstructing someone else's attempt to assess the worth of UPO's community services. But I still felt badly shaken, and in the journals I questioned my direction (*"Where do these feelings of desire for fame come from? Why are they so hard to give up?"*), my habits (*"Why do I smoke? Do I need these times to ruminate? Blame myself? Feel sorry for myself?"*), and the purpose of my life itself (*"So what's the point of all this?"*).

And I wrote about the low moods, which lasted for hours, even days:

> *I am very depressed today. I feel depressed, I walk depressed, I look depressed.*
>
> *My thoughts—I am lonely, I am unhappy, I don't want to want anything, I don't want anything but to go off and cry and make a decision about what to do from day to day. The same feeling I had Sunday.*

The private notes stopped in October 1983. Today, I attach no great significance to that silence. Since childhood, I'd had different writing projects underway and would leave one temporarily to focus on another. The summer I was nine, I wrote, typed, and sold a one-page newsletter to our neighbors. I switched to playwriting in the fall. My teacher at the time, Miss Fields, allowed me to produce and direct my plays. As a teenager, I wrote a weekly column for the *Atlanta Daily World*.

At the end of 1983 and into 1984, I seemed not to have the time for a diary. I was writing other things—a newsletter at UPO, and poetry again after a hiatus of twenty years. When I'd been an undergraduate at Howard University, I started writing poems; all had been published in *The Promethean,* the undergraduate literary magazine. But I was receiving nothing but rejection slips for the new set. As my writing teacher said of one poem, "The writing works as therapy but not as art."

The poetry was a painkiller: my marriage of thirteen years had deteriorated and ended in separation in 1984. I can't honestly blame the tumor for the breakup of my first marriage, although the tumor probably had been growing for at least a decade, perhaps more. It can't have been pleasant for the children's father to notice the gradual changes in my capacity to feel joy. It can't have been pleasant living with the depressed person I was becoming. But in the years we were married, things, as they say, had happened. I tended to think that some of the turmoil stemmed from his stint in Vietnam; I know of few veterans of that war who emerged unscathed. The split was friendly; we agreed to be good parents for our daughters.

One night amid the breakup, I saw an angel. I wrote about the visitation for my writing class. "Assurance," I called it.

I was certainly not expecting an angel, but one came to me
anyway. She visited briefly early one morning. I was going
through one more of many sleepless nights, and left my bed to
try the loveseat in my study. Like many women of thirty-five,
I was in conflict. My marriage, my job, my identity, my goals—
all were questions. I could hear no voice that was mine, only the
ceaseless babble of all the voices I'd ever heard.

They had badgered me constantly that night. As I lay on the sofa, I whispered, "Go away, leave me alone." Finally, I felt myself drifting. . . .

Until one of my girls woke me up. She touched my foot, which was hanging over one end of the loveseat.

"Alana?" I called. No answer. I called her twin. "Kali?" Still no answer.

I opened my eyes more fully and looked at this child, this presence. I saw no face or, at least, no features that I recognized. Her gown, a soft white, shone but not brightly. I touched her with my big toe. She was there. I did not speak anymore.

Nor did she ever utter words. But I got the message.

Everything is all right. She vanished. The babble ceased. I felt secure and serene.

That message became my touchstone when I was anxious or confused.

※

That same year I followed the Jesse Jackson and Charles Murray fortunes in the news; it seemed to me that one or the other was always making headlines in 1984. When Jackson ran for president that year, the press called me for comments on the PUSH/Excel program. I had none, but felt both amused and amazed to think someone I had been acquainted with was running for the highest office in the country.

Murray had become a major conservative thinker in 1984, when *Losing Ground* was published. I had known that he was writing it; he conceived it at AIR, and tossed around ideas with staff who gathered in his office after the workday. He called me once with a question about W. E. B. Du Bois and sent me a footnote, deleted from the final galleys, in which my name was mentioned. In the text, Murray had made disparaging remarks about the work of black social scientists; in the outtake, I had been cited as an exception. I have kept that curious note as a reminder of how easily evidence of competence in African Americans can disappear, while the confirming instances of inadequacy survive the editorial pen.

✖

When I resumed my private notes in August 1984, I filled as many as eight pages per day with reflections on relationships with my daughters, co-workers, and male friends (I'd begun to date) and with attempts to define some sort of ambition that would allow me finally to make my mark. I compiled lists regularly: things to do, things I had done, books and essays to write. I wrote about my divorce, which was final in January 1985. One day in February, I got the children to bed, sat down at the kitchen table, and wrote the first chapter of a novel that would appear in the journals for the next nine years. The title: *Girl Under Glass*. It was about a woman named Lene, whose little girl had witnessed the shooting of a teenager who Lene loved as a brother. Lene lived in Washington, D.C., on a street that resembled my own, and she worked in a neighborhood center much like the ones that UPO administered. After the shooting she fled to the suburbs. I, too, had run away. After a series of break-ins, I left the three-story Victorian that my children loved to roam for a new colonial with aluminum siding in one of Washington's suburbs. The story of Lene lost its momentum after I moved, and I started writing a book about Jocelyn, a sleuth who unearthed sinister family secrets.

But I hid the state of my mental health from the journals. I had seen a psychotherapist for a few months as my first marriage was ending and resumed treatment with a second person in 1986. I consulted the therapist because things were worrying me: a move to a new house and the financial burdens that moving would bring; my relationship with the man I would soon marry. The therapist suggested that I could not address problems of living until I had a floor—medication—under me. I resisted the notion for months, but just talking about my problems did little good. I felt as if I were always climbing up the sides of a dark hole, a lead weight tied to my ankles. In September 1986, four months before I married for the second time, I went to a psychiatrist said to have impeccable credentials. His diagnosis: depression.

I had never been to a psychiatrist before, but because he was a medical doctor, I expected to see stethoscopes, blood pressure cuffs, and that sort of thing in a white or pale green surrounding. Instead, the office overflowed with books and looked as someone's slightly shabby living room might. He took a long verbal history. I told him about the angel—my rational and intuitive selves were at war over what the experience represented. Was it mystical or a by-product of my depression, I asked. The psychiatrist said it was neither; it was a hypnagogic hallucination, a graphic dream that occurs as you're falling asleep.

I remember being surprised that he didn't give me a physical exam or require that I get one. He prescribed an antidepressant, Vivactyl.

The psychiatrist warned me of possible side effects, which did indeed appear. The videotape of my wedding shows two of them. In the tape I am well on the way to twenty-five pounds of extra weight and I am constantly licking my lips from dry mouth. In the following months, my depression didn't lift; I had crying spells, and I was constantly anxious. When I continued to show no signs of improvement, the psychiatrist added lithium, used to treat manic-depressive illness.

I hid my depression from all but a handful of people. I was embarrassed and feared that I might be viewed suspiciously on my job, which by then—the year was 1987—was Director of Planning for the community action agency in Fairfax County, Virginia. I continued to be depressed, but managed to mask it when I went for a job interview in 1988 at Johns Hopkins. I talked about the community's role in youth development, but the Hopkins staff seemed more eager to talk about the study I'd conducted with Murray and Jackson.

From 1989 on, the personal entries in my journal reflected a depression that deepened rather than lifted, as I'd hoped:

There is no magic. No God. No hope. I do not believe in anything anymore not love not God not brighter days or social science research have hit rock bottom am crying do not believe in pills, psychotherapy, writing fiction we all die anyway. I am a piece of dead shit.

I tried to cope with the depression:

I must surround myself daily with things, thoughts, relations that inspire, not drag me down.

Nature tapes—like the ones in the country store
Green plants in my window at work
Writing in my diary.

Despite my emotional problems, my intellectual functioning seemed to be normal. I had few journal entries in 1990; I'd been writing four research articles. All were published the following year.

⚜

I remained on lithium until sometime in the fall of 1990. Months before, the psychiatrist had said I could discontinue the Vivactyl and could take the lithium as needed. I don't recall now whether I consulted him before I stopped taking the lithium altogether; taking it as needed hadn't seemed to make a difference. I still had to work hard to have a mildly pleasant time, especially at my work as a mom. My stepson, Kobie, was living with us, and with three teenagers roughly the same age, motherhood became a triple challenge. I was with them most of the time when I wasn't at work. In addition to his regular job at a university counseling center, my husband had started a private psychotherapy practice and was at his office in Washington much of the time. Shopping, cleaning, cooking, yard work, and monitoring homework all fell to my domain. The hard work of being a parent, however, had its rewards: my children were becoming independent, sensitive, and at times boisterous and outgoing teenagers. Our house, a block from the high school they attended, was the after-school choice for their friends, and they did homework, watched Oprah and the soaps, and raided the refrigerator for leftovers.

But again I had lost the desire and energy to write poetry. My novel was stalled. I felt estranged from old friends, and my husband and I were becoming silent partners. I was constantly in motion, fueled by the scheduled demands of children, spouse, Hopkins, community, and house. I was still depressed, still telling myself, "Saundra, you have it all. Why can't you just pull yourself together and get on with it?" In December of 1990, I sought help from yet another psychotherapist.

※

"*Happy New Year!*" I had written in my journal. I started 1991 without medication for the first time in three years. I was pleased with the handful of sessions I had with Maureen, my new therapist, and I felt rested after the holidays. But on January 3, I recorded the first of some puzzling physical symptoms:

Tried to go to work today but turned around on I-70 because I felt faint. Makes me appreciate my usual vigor and good health. One thing about being sick. It makes you set priorities.

The feelings of faintness had been brief; I was back at work the next day.

I was more determined than ever to fight the depression, which hadn't gone anywhere, and throughout 1991 and 1992, I used my journals as the battlefield. I added self-praise for uplift ("*Congratulations Saundra! Look at what you've achieved. Tomorrow you're going to a conference on resilience with the President of the W. T. Grant Foundation. You will be with the giants in the resilience field. Way to go!*"); wrote little plays with "anxiety" in one role and me in the other; recorded accounts of specific efforts I made on a given day to cope emotionally (*"went to therapy, talked to mom"*), physically (*"had a check-up; thyroid problem?"*), spiritually (*"read a meditation"*), and mentally (*"gave this part a well-deserved rest"*); and described what made me feel grateful:

> *Some lovely moments since the last entry. Tonight, a potluck with my writers' group. Last week—in the kitchen with the girls. I was eating watermelon & Alana came in and said "Thick pink imperial slices." She then read to Kali and me the poem by John Tobias in which those lines appeared. A good moment, "unicorns become possible again" as another line in the poem says.*

But the depression was relentless, and I wrote about crying spells more and more frequently. An added twist was that they had become public: in a furniture store, at the airport, in my writers' groups. I felt I had good reason to cry. My second marriage was over. Alana and I had moved in July 1992, a month after Kobie graduated from high school and Kali decided to skip her senior year and enroll at Hopkins in the fall. The entries from July and August summed up my concerns, which were mostly about the children and the breakup of the marriage.

I think now that the tumor troubled the marriage at every turn. I had made major decisions—to court, to marry, to separate—and countless other choices in between. But I know the tumor wasn't the sole cause of the breakup; my husband and I had, as the separation agreement says, many "disputes and unhappy differences." We had been unable to reconcile them. In dreams I recorded in my journals, I am always trying to get away—in an airplane, in my car, on foot.

I felt relieved after the separation; I began to write affirmations ("I *am worthy. I am a child of God"*) and nearly every day something good about my life:

> *I went to Inverness last Monday. God's country. Stayed in a lovely inn that opened onto a stream and a small meadow with deer. The mountains were in the distance. I slept with the windows open so I could see those mountains when I woke up.*

I wrote one or two poems and made some progress on the novels. I worried about Alana; she played varsity soccer and was undergoing tests for a possible brain injury she received while practicing. Fortunately, the tests were negative. And I fretted about money; my debt was mounting. Still, by the end of August 1992, I was able to write:

> *On the way home from the party, I realized that I could be very happy—I am happy—single with good friends & interesting activities—like antiquing, looking for black dolls, china, old prints & other goodies.*

And in September:

> *I am going to affirm that all things are working together for the highest good of all concerned. I have a sense of her—the person I am becoming. She is unselfish, conscious, but aware of reality, the now & responsive to it, fully engaged and enjoying life. I hope I can become her.*

I still cried and felt depressed and fatigued. Two physical symptoms had emerged: rapid heartbeat and tingling in my left arm. I recorded these symptoms infrequently. Although they occurred only three or four times in 1992 and 1993, they frightened me. Each time I'd been driving and had no memory of the circumstances that triggered them. I usually had to pull off the road and wait for things to calm down. Drinking a glass of water helped. My doctor had suspected a thyroid problem, but my tests had been within the normal range.

⚒

The dreamer in me had known something was up. I'd awakened, frightened, one morning in April 1993 and written in my journal:

Dream. I am standing next to a black, middle-aged man (doctor). We're waiting to review brain X-rays for K—although she wasn't there when the pictures were taken.

And a few days later, on April 27:

I just got up at 4:45 after turning in bed for two hrs & wrote. I must write fiction or poetry at every opportunity—replace the internal useless obsessions (mad thoughts running scared in my brain)—it feels full.

After that, a shift. There were no more poems. I wrote the last one in the first days of April. It was a sad poem about two would-be lovers, telling their separate tales of lost battles.

I made fewer and fewer lists, as if I were losing awareness of where I had been in the immediate past and what I wanted to do in the future.

I no longer kept accounts of my actions in spiritual and other areas. Instead, I had begun to record predictions from *The I Ching*, an ancient Chinese text used for divination and meditation on major changes in life.

The reflections, navel-gazing, and questions decreased. I wrote fewer pages. Description was sparse. My handwriting became fainter, sometimes illegible, with little spikes and peaks, unlike the flowing cursive that I had mastered in the third grade and had used ever since. I misspelled simple nouns. I inserted extra digits in dates.

In 1994 I wrote about thirty entries only. I had been actively searching for a teaching position, but I recorded nothing about the searches and job talks I had. I wrote not one word about the divorce proceedings, which were contentious, nor had I said anything about the memory losses, the aphasic episode that ended in a trip to the emergency room, or the family reunion.

Of the entries that I did write, most were only a few lines long. I was depressed (*"Have been up most of the night crying"*). I was obsessed with my new responsibilities at UM. On October 1, 1994, I'd written an affirmation, *"I am a good teacher,"* ten times.

※

What had I known and when and how had I known it? I can't answer these questions with certainty, but by the last months of 1994, I knew I could no longer use my writing. I had lost the capacity to feel the mind, the heart, and the hand work together. The tumor was silent tissue, beyond words, nourished by a nightmarish code that permeated every cell in my body. The brainless spirit, the tumor, was gaining ground.

Witnesses

I stopped dreaming sometime during the fall of 1994. Or maybe I couldn't remember my dreams long enough for them to inspire me or to haunt me. Waking life had a floating, gossamer haze, except when I stepped into the classroom. There, everything suddenly was vivid, sharp, terrifying. A nightmare.

I added a third course to my schedule. The course was taught by a team representing three state institutions. We met for class in Baltimore; the students were full-time teachers in a master's degree program. When my daughters visited on weekends, we sat around the kitchen table and discussed my shortcomings as a teacher. It became a ritual.

I would say: "I am boring, can't keep my students' attention. They walk out at the break or read *The Diamondback* (the UM student newspaper) right in front of me. I can't answer questions sometimes. I can't remember my students' names."

"Mom, people read *The Diamondback* in some of my classes. Some of my professors are boring." This was the voice of Alana, a sophomore at UM. She had been elected to county and statewide student governing boards and had years of participation as a student and a staff member of the Maryland Leadership Workshops. "You have to mix it up. Try some cooperative learning groups. You show films— get some that are up-to-date. Some of your students grew up with MTV."

Kali was a junior at Hopkins. Kali would wear me down with long, trenchant arguments about the relative merits of large and small universities and the implications for student learning. She'd wind up with something like, "Mom, chill. You've been doing research and now you're teaching. You can't be doing everything wrong."

Despite repeated rounds of this discussion, my daughters never complained. The three of us never attributed my uncertain performance to physical symptoms I was having, symptoms that seemed to be multiplying and making themselves known in the midst of my class activities. One of my students, who worked in an optometrist's office, told me later that I removed my glasses often, saying that things looked blurry. She tried some minor adjustments to the frames. The glasses were fairly new. I had shifted to lineless bifocals and thought I was having difficulty adjusting to the dual lens.

Another time I asked a student, "Well, what are you doing here?" when she mentioned one day in class that she had a migraine. I told her that I had headaches all the time, and she said that I often held my head as if in pain. But I don't recall the headaches. What I remember feeling was a stuffiness, a floating pressure—the kind you have when you get a head cold. I noticed it most in the evenings and must have taken medicines that relieved it.

After I came home from the hospital, I found my medicine cabinet filled with half-empty bottles of aspirin and other pain-killers. That was odd. Most of my life I'd kept few medications around the house—my standard first-aid kit was aspirin, something for stomach-aches, a box of bandages, maybe some cough syrup.

Fortunately, most of the symptoms didn't last too long. I willed myself to appear well, and as October passed, I thought that I was responding more rapidly to students' questions and managing to speak in paragraphs without losing words along the way. I managed to restrict my response to colleagues' "How're you doing?" to "Pretty well, thanks, and you?"

※

On the last Saturday of October, I felt well enough to go with my friend Lisa to see Derek Walcott's *The Odyssey,* at Arena Stage in Washington. When the house lights came up, Lisa and I walked to her car. The ride back took us along Constitution Avenue, which runs alongside the Mall with the Smithsonian Institution and the Washington Monument to the left and the White House to the right. Lisa and I talked about how much we had enjoyed the evening, but I thought I should critique the performance. At that moment my mind would not, probably could not, begin to form abstractions. "You don't have to analyze it," Lisa said. "Just feel it." In fact, my experience of the play had been in the pleasures of the senses: I remembered the cadences of Telemachus, Penelope, and the narrator "Blind" Billy Blue; the Calypso accents of the music; the hot pink gauze dresses worn by the women in Circe's brothel. Ordinary delight had replaced the uncontrollable emotions and sensations I had experienced just the week before, after I'd visited the primary care physician.

Months later, I read the play because I could not remember even a single phrase. In the final scene, Odysseus's homecoming, Penelope says to him, "The sea is quiet and all your trials are done." Perhaps during the performance my nervous system had picked up this line, stored it directly in my brain, and produced whatever effect affirmations have.

Two weeks later on November 12, I managed another event without a major mishap. *I Hear a Symphony: African Americans Celebrate Love*, the book in which my poem "War Stories" had been published, was introduced in the Washington area. One of the editors called to give me a list of stops on the book tour that I could attend. I chose the last location, the Hirshhorn Museum at the Smithsonian, because I wanted to be rested for the occasion.

As I sat in the darkened auditorium, I crossed my fingers; I did not want the editors to recognize me. I did not want to speak. After the formal presentations, a few people asked me to autograph my poem. I wrote slowly, willing my mind to stay in there and not go wandering, wordless, leaving my fingers limp and unable to hold the pen.

My daughters and I had Thanksgiving dinner with friends. Kali and Alana had come for the holidays, only to find the refrigerator empty. Kali, who produced gourmet meals, was particularly appalled. "Mom, what have you been eating? Everything is dried up or sour." I didn't mention it, but I seemed to have lost the taste for food, and had given up going to the grocery store, enduring the check-out lines, and fighting the fatigue that accompanied me as I moved down one aisle and up the next. I was living on a diet of fast food. But even the fast foods were a problem. After classes, I would go to the drive-through, select a hamburger, salad, and a drink and then forget the order by the time I had to yell into the loudspeakers. I'd end up paying for milk and French fries or whatever I remembered to say. At some point, I gave up the drive-through and went inside. I could manage to give my order while I kept my eyes on the menu board, but I couldn't always get out the words.

Nor, it seemed, could I rely on other parts of my body. At the end of November, I went to a dance. I felt OK that evening, but to conserve energy I stood back and watched others perform. I stepped out and joined them for a line dance that I had done for years and enjoyed. But when the group shuffled to the right, I went left. I forgot to turn at the appropriate time and bumped into someone else. My legs felt like heavy rubber. Embarrassed and puzzled, I left the dance floor.

※

I had another aphasic episode when the daylight hours were very short, the weather was cold enough for heavy coats, and the semester was ending. I don't remember details. My colleague Jamie, a developmental psychologist, wrote what she witnessed that day when I lost my words:

> It was after work one day. Almost everyone had left the department—but Saundra and I had both just finished teaching for the day. We started talking—I don't exactly know what about. We were, at one point, discussing how it was going here at Maryland for Saundra—given it was her first year. Our conversation started in the department entrance. I think Saundra was getting

somewhat upset—or maybe frustrated at her speech. I followed her into her office and we resumed our conversation.

Saundra was telling me that she had not been doing well. On top of the load she'd been given for this first semester at Maryland—including [meetings] and teaching in Baltimore—she started to tell me about a lot of the outside stressors which she was then experiencing. These included going through a divorce, both daughters living away from home—change of job and unfamiliarity in everything around her. She did say she had been "depressed" and was seeing a therapist—of whom she was very fond and trusting.

Throughout the conversation, Saundra experienced frequent inability to talk. She would be in the middle of saying something, or about to embark on a sentence, and nothing would come out. At these times, Saundra closed her eyes and stayed or made herself quite calm, giving herself time and then trying again. The "lost voice" was not a consequence of extreme emotional upset, as when someone is crying too hard to talk. Saundra was quite composed and not crying as these attempts to talk failed her. She had said that she'd recently seen a physician to eliminate a physical cause for her current psychological and speech problems.

I had never witnessed what Saundra was experiencing. A depressed person may have difficulty talking about a particular topic, may have too little energy to feel like talking, or may talk about other topics to avoid the difficult emotions. Saundra was trying to communicate and her speech would not come. She was very frustrated and very puzzled by this strange and debilitating experience.

I left Saundra's office very worried about her—but not understanding there was a physical cause. I felt reassured that she had a current therapist and that she'd consulted with medical doctors to rule out a physical cause. I was still left with the feeling that Saundra was at a very dark and lonely place, very depressed; a place that it would be a hard battle to return from.

✂

My parents came to Maryland that Christmas, although my father was scheduled to have eye surgery the following month. I'd told them I was simply too exhausted to go to Atlanta for the holidays. I managed to decorate the house: poinsettias in every room, a Douglas fir in the living room, candles on the tables, and a large wreath on the front door.

The symptoms seemed to have abated. We listened to Christmas albums: Nat King Cole, Kiri Te Kanawa, The Temptations. The "posse"—my daughters' friends from high school—dropped by two or three times, exchanged gifts, and hung out with the family. My mother picked a wing chair in the living room and settled there each evening to read and crochet while my dad made little repairs around the house. We opened gifts on Christmas morning and feasted on cornish hens at dinner.

My mother said she knew something was wrong when one day after Christmas I burst into tears about paying a bill for some repairs someone was making in our bathroom.

Another day Kali and my father were cutting vegetables while I made the base for bean soup. She started to pour in the onions. I screamed, "You don't put the onions in first. The celery goes in first. And the chunks are too big. You just never listen to me. You and Alana don't respect me. You two don't like me."

Other than those outbursts, and my anxiety about the stack of final papers I had to finish by the first week of the coming year, Christmas was a happy time. Fran, my oldest and dearest friend, who lives in Detroit, sent gifts to Alana and Kali. On a card she'd written, "Call if there's a crisis with your mother."

My parents returned to Atlanta on December 29. Alana and Kali slept in the mornings and spent afternoons and evenings out with friends. I graded papers and slept, worked on a report and slept. One day, I screamed at the girls when they hadn't awakened me to take a phone call. "Mom," Alana said, "you told us you didn't want to be disturbed." After I shouted at them when they charged fifteen dollars on a credit card, they told their father they were worried that I was having a nervous breakdown: "Mom's finally lost it."

※

Maureen, my therapist, thought I was unstable and considered putting me in the hospital. Starting on December 30 and continuing for about two weeks, she made notes of my calls and visits. I used her dates and my calendar to construct a chronology, but the feelings and events come from my memory.

December 30. I go to the kitchen, open a drawer, take out a knife. I place the knife on a vein. I put the knife back in the drawer. If I kill myself, my daughters won't get my insurance. I take two Ativan and call Maureen. I tell her I don't think the thoughts of suicide are dangerous. She wants me to call anytime when I feel that way again.

Earlier that evening, I'd gone to the first of two parties to which I'd been invited. When I arrived, I tried to say something pleasant, but instead started crying. The hostess led me to a room upstairs, but I couldn't stop. I apologized and left. I didn't go to the second party. Even if I'd been able to go, I'd forgotten how to get there.

January 2, 1995. I turn in the grades for two of my courses and go to therapy. I tell Maureen I don't want to live.

January 7, 1995. A terrible day. The third course I am teaching meets in Baltimore for the final examination. It is an assessment of student portfolios. One group presents some "hands-on" exercises in which other students and the instructors have to participate. One exercise, designed for elementary school children, is a simple task involving word associations. I fail to get even one of the associations correct within the time allotted for the entire task.

January 9, 1995. I go to therapy and once again, I struggle with thoughts of suicide. Later that day, I call Maureen, disappointed over a six-week courtship that ended abruptly.

January 11, 1995. I see Maureen. She thinks I am in a "much better place" with the end of the courtship and "have a handle" on suicidal feelings. I say I will call her if they recur.

The suicidal thoughts vanish. I go about my work at the two universities during the week, feeling like my old self. On January 14, I go to the market for food. Kali is coming home for the weekend. I am talking on the phone to a friend when I have my final blackout.

Scholar, mother, wife, friend. Western culture gave me these roles, complete with a lifetime of scripts, canned, neatly stacked on the shelf, and ready for distribution. Word for word, deed by deed, I'd rehearsed my lines for nearly half a century, departing from my prescribed part only in those rare times when I'd felt strong, in control, safe. In *Brain Repair,* neuroscientists ask, "What does a lifetime of establishing 'habits' do to the ability to compensate for brain-injury—especially when one considers all of the cultural and social events that influence what we learn and remember?"[1] Such was the power of habits and roles that I have passed for normal, innocently deceiving loved ones, colleagues, physicians, and just about everyone else, even as my mind forgot its routine functions, and in the process, forgot me as well.

� On Meyer Nine

"Don't worry," the nurse says. "I won't leave you until you're all checked in at the hospital." I think he is holding my hand. I seem to be aware of looking into his eyes; and moments later aware of the equipment in the ambulance; still later of rolling to a standstill, then rolling through an entry. Acute triage, a sign says. Does the gurney stop at the desk, pause perhaps, before they wheel me to a curtained cubicle? "I am Dr. Eric Oshiro." He is the neurosurgeon who admits me to Johns Hopkins Hospital, but I don't recall what he says or does next. The nurse lingers. I think he is keeping his promise. I am calm. He leaves. I am wheeled on a gurney through corridors and onto an elevator. It stops. We are on the top floor of the building, Meyer Nine, the floor for neurosurgical patients. It is my home for the next twelve days.

✻

On the night of January 14, I was assigned to Room 919, a single room. Nearly all the rooms on Meyer Nine are singles. Somewhere between the Hopkins emergency room and my room, someone removed my street clothes and dressed me in a hospital gown. A nurse introduced herself as the night nurse. She held a small, pleated paper cup filled with several pills.

I heard her voice and someone walking in the hallway. I remember the bed with its white sheets and blanket, the table on wheels, the chair in the corner, the long window on one wall, covered with curtains in a pale green, lavender, and pink plaid. On the chest next to the bed, there was a rose plastic cup and pitcher. I put the pills in my mouth and tasted just a hint of pure chemical as they rested at the back of my tongue before I gulped water and pills down my throat.

I went to sleep without a thought. It was the first time in decades that I hadn't said even a quick prayer. I couldn't. My brain was recording impressions from the world, but it had stopped putting words together or adding numbers or even remembering that I was Saundra and I was in this hospital because I had a brain tumor.

That night I woke up and wandered into the hallway where a short man dressed in a hospital uniform was walking. "You're new?" he asked. I said nothing. "You look scared," he continued. "Tell you what. I know somebody who would be real good for you to meet. He's a patient. Don't worry. Go get some rest. I'll hook you up."

�֎

Early Sunday morning, someone wheels me to a room with a large white cylinder in it. I am tired and sleepy and only manage to say "whatever" after the technician explains that the neurosurgeon has ordered scans of my brain. I am vaguely aware of being assisted to a narrow cot and asked to lie flat on my back and not move. I doze.

The loud knocks rouse me. I see only a white steel dome above my head and to the right and the left. A blanket covers my prone body. Again, loud metallic knocks. I inhale, let a small stream of air pass through my nostrils.

I am sliding. I leave the place where I am confined through a hole, feet first. The light is sterile and bright. I tremble in the cool air. A voice says, "Sit up slowly." Later, I learn that I've had a brain scan by a sophisticated method known as magnetic resonance imaging, or MRI. The report says, "There is a 6 cm ¥ 6 cm ¥ 5.5 cm extra-axial mass." The tumor.

As I am wheeled back to my floor, I feel a pulse inside my head, but at least I can think about it being there. Everyone and everything is strange. I know I am in a hospital. I wonder whether my daughters know I'm here. My parents? My friends?

Even in my mental murk, I am aware of moving through bright, colorful corridors that have no discernible vanishing points. There is a hum of human voices and big machines. It comes from the spaces behind doors that are affixed with the paperwork of patients or the labels of physicians and medical departments.

᠅

The Johns Hopkins hospital is as unlike the hospital of my childhood as the Wright brothers' aircraft is from a jumbo jet. My family had used Harris Memorial Hospital, a renovated one-story house on West Hunter Street (since renamed Martin Luther King Jr. Avenue). Ever since I could remember and before, West Hunter was one of several sites of thriving black businesses: Amos Drug Store (home of the best cherry cokes), Paschal's restaurant and motel,

Adams' photography studio, the bank, and Bronner Brothers hair supply. Harris itself was owned by the Harris family; one of the sisters was the organist at Friendship Baptist, the church I had attended nearly every Sunday. I was born at Harris, as were my sister, Pat, and brother, Hal. My mother had major surgery there on two occasions. At Christmas, our Girl Scout troop took gifts to the small patients in the children's ward. We sang carols and tried to be cheerful, but we avoided talking with each other when we walked back to our school a few blocks away. My own childhood home was only a ten-minute walk from Harris, which seemed more like a benign extension of our family dwelling than a sterile institution.

Except for two or three trips to the emergency room, I'd had only one hospital stay. When I gave birth to Kali and Alana, I'd had a Caesarean section, developed an infection, and was hospitalized for seven days. The year was 1975; I watched Arthur Ashe win Wimbledon as I tried to nurse the twins. The girls were beautiful and had good scores on all the indices the pediatrician used.

※

The elevator doors closed; we were going up to Meyer Nine. My stomach lurched the way it did when an airplane took off. I traveled by myself for business frequently, and when I flew, I feared that if the plane crashed, I would die alone.

Kali and Barbara had wanted to accompany me in the ambulance. They were told they couldn't do that, and besides, I would arrive at the hospital after visiting hours.

Kali and Alana were nineteen. I've heard their story about how they handled the "brain explosion," as Alana calls it. They notified my parents and sister, my friend Fran, and other people close to me. They spent Saturday night with their "Grandma Rosa" Murray, who comforted them with homemade vegetable soup. Kathy Murray, their aunt who is a pediatrician at Children's Hospital in Washington, questioned them about my symptoms and said she would do what she could to get information. Alana assumed the role of family spokesperson. My daughters believed that I would survive and did not show any fear in my presence.

After the first night, I was rarely alone. On Sunday morning before visiting hours, the man I'd seen in the hallway came into my room. "I said I'd hook you up. This is Ted. Gotta go. I'll check in on you later." Ted was middle-aged; his skull was bandaged. He sat by my bed, asked why I was there, and told me not to be afraid, that God would take care of me. He prayed with me, said he had cancer, and would be going home later in the week, but he'd stop by later in the day with his minister.

I answered lots of phone calls that morning: my daughters, Barbara, my neighbors. Maureen's notes record that I called her and told her I had a brain tumor. With the help of a nurse, who dialed the number for me, I called my parents to tell them about my illness. I have no recollection of the conversation, but my father taped the call. In it, I was lucid some of the time, correctly ascribing my depression to the tumor, which I referred to as a growth. I was very concerned about getting back to work; my parents encouraged me not to worry about that. Because my father had had an eye operation the very week my tumor was diagnosed, my mother said she would come after my surgery and stay with me for as long as it took me to get better. As the conversation continued, my comments became downright bizarre.

It seemed as if I lost focus or could not understand my parents' questions. When my dad asked whether I would be able to climb stairs after the operation, I replied, "Oh. I think that going upstairs would be satisfactory. I just think it was too many people there before."

※

During visiting hours, Kali, Alana, and Barbara came with a big suitcase of my personal items: gowns, books, tapes, cosmetics, and teddy bears. My neighbors, Marcia and Suellen, came that evening. Ted and his minister dropped by. We held hands and prayed together.

After that, the people and days merged into the rhythms of the hospital: visits from family and friends; visits from nurses bearing medicines, taking blood; and visits from cafeteria staff with food. Ted returned and brought the first gifts: a calendar of inspirational quotes and a small arrangement of roses in a pink flowerpot. The roses faded before I left the hospital, but I have kept the container planted with silk flowers as a reminder of Ted's kindness. He was discharged before I learned his last name and address.

The neurosurgical residents came to see me early each day, before breakfast. I have never been a morning person; I do my best work beginning around three in the afternoon and into the night. In my drugged state, it was all I could do to lift my head from the pillow, let alone smile, when the doctors, friendly and heavy-footed, came as a little herd into the room. The exam was brief, simply a few questions and instructions: Where are you? Why are you here? What day is it? Smile. Extend your arms and pretend you're holding a pizza. Say, "No ifs, ands, or buts."

Much of the time, my thinking seemed clear, if slow, and I felt relatively calm. I suppose the drugs had something to do with my outlook. When I was admitted, I was put on a regimen of dexamethasone (Decadron), a powerful steroid to reduce the intense swelling of my brain; phenytoin (Dilantin), to prevent seizures; and ranitidine (Zantac), to decrease stomach distress. I also continued to take the Ativan and hormones. I recognized my friends, who said I talked about my condition in a detached, clinical way. "You weren't there," said one friend. With another friend, I readily remembered key people in my professional networks so that he could contact them; soon, I received dozens of cards, notes, long-distance calls, and gifts of flowers, books, plants, and candy.

Kathy, my daughters' aunt, offered to confer with my doctors and convey the information about the prognosis and procedures to my family. Fran said she would help with Alana's school expenses. One friend called every night before the surgery and sang to me: "He's a God you can't hurry. . . . He may not come when you want Him, But when He comes He's right on time." Yet another friend read Second Timothy, chapter seven, every night. She said she had to fish around for it and thought it was a godsend: "For God hath not given us the spirit of fear; but of power, and of love, and of a sound mind." Jim, Barbara's husband and a professor in my department, phoned to say that my colleagues would be covering my classes. One of my Hopkins friends assisted Kali with registration.

At first I couldn't understand all the kindness, the prayers, the gentle words of hope. I'd felt so alone in the months before the diagnosis, as if each person with whom I'd come in contact had seen only little parts or fleeting moments of me. I eventually relaxed in the love and friendship; I sensed the support was just as much for them as it was for me. I saw in their eyes the helplessness, the vulnerability, the knowledge that, there, but for the grace of God. . . .

※

One day, Dr. Oshiro told me that he was bringing in another neurosurgeon, Dr. Rafael Tamargo, who was particularly skilled at removing the kind of tumor they suspected I had. They came to my room to talk with me and to answer questions that I'd written in a faint, spidery handwriting on a little pad that a friend had given me.

Can I exchange picture of my MRIs and other things with a
    physician outside of this hospital?
Is there possibility that I can do without an operation?
What time is the standard time for recovery (with/without) the
    time spent in the hospital?
When could I have an operation?
When I get through the recovery period, I'll be halfway through
    a semester. Should I make arrangements?
When would I have to exercise my power of attorney?

As the questions show, I was confused about details.

The doctors gave me direct answers. Kathy was welcome to information about my case. I would die without surgery, which was scheduled for Thursday, January 19, five days after I'd been admitted; radiation and chemotherapy could not be used until the tumor was removed. I should identify someone to whom I would give power of attorney.

I don't remember the answers to other questions, but if there had been a part of me that anticipated the worst, there was a part that expected and affirmed the best. That part grew stronger as I received word that a great many people were praying for my recovery and, in some cases, had asked their church congregations to remember me in their prayers. No one who visited revealed the fear that I would die, and it seldom occurred to me that I could be seeing or hearing my family, friends, and colleagues for the last time. I thought there was a slim chance that I could die, but more often I thought I would survive with all my powers intact. I did not yet understand how diminished I had become.

I was determined to do everything I could to live. Faced with the option of death if I did not undergo the operation, the suicidal thoughts I'd had prior to the diagnosis never entered my mind. When I was tempted to think about what was happening and why I was there, I studied the colors and shapes of the plants and flowers that were arranged in the window that stretched the length of one wall, listened to tapes of Aretha, Mozart, Bonnie Raitt, or sang to myself the refrain from a song I learned in the choir in elementary school: "I love life. I want to live. I love life."

✼

I did little to put my affairs in order. My children were the beneficiaries of my estate. With my life insurance and my retirement fund, there would be enough for them to pay off the mortgage if they chose to, and to pay for the rest of their education. I decided not to give anyone power of attorney, and no one urged me to do that. A sign of hope? Or denial? I think it was both, plus the faith that I'd had since I was a small child in the Cradle Room of Friendship Baptist Church, where I'd clutched a tiny card with a picture of Jesus on the front and a short Bible verse on the back. My adult faith was a simple collage of rituals and values that I'd pieced together from visits to different churches and temples, readings of religious and philosophical texts, and music—spirituals, Protestant hymns, Buddhist chants, masses, and oratorios. Cutting through this assemblage was a sign in blue neon that had been installed near the ceiling in Friendship's sanctuary. The sign asked, "What think ye of Christ?" As a little girl, I'd had plenty of Sundays to ponder that question. It flashed through my mind many times again as the day of the operation approached.

A day or two before the operation the anesthesiologist came by to get some information on my health. Despite the years of symptoms from the tumor, I'd had no major or minor health complaints. I seldom had colds or flu; I ate healthy food. Exercise had been hit-or-miss; I took ballet and modern dance before and shortly after my children were born; when they were five, we took a mother and daughter tap dance class at the Y; and thereafter I crunched and burned first to a Jane Fonda record and later to her videos or any fitness show that happened to be on television before work.

The anesthesiologist asked questions about my history. The main one I remembered was "Do you smoke?" I said I used to, but quit about ten years ago. She thought I'd have few problems with being anesthetized for a long period of time. She said I was "young and healthy."

Wednesday, January 18, was the day before the surgery. To me it seemed pretty much like the previous three days since I had come to Meyer Nine. I talked for a long time to my parents in Atlanta. My daughters came by after classes. The calm demeanors did not deceive me; I sensed that fear and adrenaline were keeping them going.

Each one told me about her day. Alana was taking statistics and accounting; she said it was rough with the typical antics of the freshmen she supervised in the dorm, and the part-time job she had for raising spending money. Kali had been to classes, and had worked for a few hours at the education research center at Hopkins, the same one at which I worked during the summers. Before they left, they kissed me and assured me that I'd be OK; their Aunt Kathy told them that tumors like the one I had were easily operable and typically nonmalignant.

The last visitors I had that night were a colleague from UM and a friend from Hopkins. The three of us seemed giddy. I have no recollection of what we talked about, although I knew that my friend had written me a long note when I began my job at Maryland. After visiting hours, Dr. Tamargo came by and asked if I had any questions about the operation. I think I asked something like, will I regain my powers. He said, "It's in God's hands. Make sure you say your prayers. I will certainly say mine."

About 5 A.M. on the morning of the surgery, I woke up, thought about what was going to happen in a few hours, and felt my breathing become shallow and my left arm go weak and numb. Those were the signs of an imminent panic attack—I recognized them from previous bouts—but I feared a heart attack. Not trusting the call bell, I tried to calm myself, walked to the nurses' station, and told them what was happening. I was told to return to my room. They would handle everything. I managed to get back to my bed before my heart started its rapid, unrelenting pounding.

The cavalry arrived: Trae, the nurse assigned to my case, told me to take deep breaths, while her colleague started connecting me to the EKG. While the nurses worked, I had my only long moments of fear throughout the entire ordeal. I hadn't seen the Grim Reaper, or experienced my life flashing before me, or white light at the end of a tunnel. Nothing. What scared me was that I could no longer make a bargain with God. All my life I'd made such promises, contingent, of course, on God coming through for me. If only you'll help me to pass algebra, I'll do all my homework problems. If only you pull my friend through this ordeal, I promise to call her every day to check on her. Now, there were no more bargains.

Trae must have sensed something, or maybe she saw physical signs of anxiety. She held me and said, "We don't know what the future holds, but we know who holds the future." After the nurses left, I prayed for the strength for my loved ones and for me to deal with whatever came next.

※

This could be my last morning, I thought. But I was not capable of dwelling on it. Someone brought my breakfast, which I wasn't allowed to eat. The surgery was scheduled for nine. Kali came in, her loaded book bag slung between her slender shoulders. She patted my shoulder. "Mom, stop crying," she said briskly. I had not known I was. A nurse came in and told us they would be putting me into another room after the surgery. Apparently, my room, close to the nurses' station, was reserved for patients who had to be monitored frequently. I got up to gather my things, but Kali protested, "Let me, Mom." I felt like a trapped animal, frightened and wary. My questions came rapidly, in no particular order. Why did I have to move? Where's my ring? Will they shave all of my hair? Why can't my daughter eat my breakfast? When will Alana arrive? Can Kali come with me when they wheel me away? What will happen if the tumor's malignant?

Once again I was wheeled away from Meyer Nine, with Kali walking beside the gurney. Somewhere along the way, Kali left; she and Alana would meet in the waiting room with their father and some of their friends.

Later, I recognized the anesthesiologist who had evaluated me a couple of days before. With her was another anesthesiologist, a man. They were the last two people I saw. My eyes closed and my fear was gone; I rested in invisible arms.

After the operation, my daughters told me that Dr. Tamargo and Dr. Oshiro had burst into the waiting room "like teammates who'd won the Superbowl." I had survived the operation, the doctors thought they had completely removed the tumor, and it was not malignant.

I also had a big head. The girls saw me right after the operation. "You looked awful, Mom," Kali said. "We were really worried because your head was all swollen, the size of a football." Alana had said, "You were crying even though you were unconscious. We thought you were in pain." The nurses reassured them; the brain feels no pain. Later, Dr. Tamargo told me that the eyes can become irritated during surgery. Tears accumulate and afterward, the cornea drains.

The nurses urged the girls to talk to me and tell me that I was OK. Soon I was in intensive care.

As I regain consciousness, I try to ask the question I feel. Am I alive? The nurse says I'm just fine. I want water. The nurse says they have to limit my intake of liquids because of swelling of the brain. She says she needs to check on another patient, but I'm hooked to a monitor that will signal if I thump my hand against the bed.

I doze off only to reawaken to scratchy sounds from the radio. I know bad rock music when I hear it. I motioned for the nurse and mumbled, then grimaced. She laughed and asked if I wanted to hear classical music. I have no idea what I did to tell her yes, but she changed the station. "A woman after my own heart," she said. I fell asleep to the sounds of French horns and strings.

I came to when they gave me a blood transfusion. A question was forming in my mind, but I couldn't hold onto it. Later, a rolling sensation awakened me. I was wheeled through the halls once more, this time back to Meyer Nine. I was fully awake two days later. My sister Pat sat by my bed, crying and holding my hand. "They really cut your head open," she said. "I didn't believe it, but now I see for myself."

Fran's daughter sat on the bed; she had sneaked her infant son past the nurses' station and rocked him so he would stay quiet. Alana and Kali were in the room. I had the urge to comb my hair. "Hand me the instrument that's opposite a comb," I said slowly. I could speak! Only I didn't know the word for brush. And my head was partially bald and covered by a large white bandage. I didn't need that elusive word.

My sister helped me into my pink terry-cloth robe, and we walked arm in arm to the nurses' station and back, the first of many steps I would have to take to reenter the world.

The next day, a Sunday, I wrote my first words, *"Health and whole-ness,"* in a blank notebook my daughters had packed.

Before the tumor I had half thoughts, half writings, half battles
After the tumor, I have wholeness, a breath, a whole breath
  my vision—wonderful vision.

The next day I started writing lists again: questions about medica-tion, names of people I needed to contact about my work responsi-bilities; items on the hospital's breakfast menu to replicate at home.

I walked to the lounge on Meyer Nine every chance I got and looked through the large plates of glass toward Fell's Point, part of the Balti-more harbor, and about fifteen blocks away from the hospital down a street named Broadway. I was sure the television show *Homicide* had filmed some episodes there. One evening I saw a copy of *Architectural Digest* on a table. I decided it was time to discover how much I could read, understand, and remember. I picked a short article from the magazine and scanned a couple of paragraphs. I recognized all the words and understood most of the ideas, but I couldn't remember a thing I'd read. I didn't know whether to feel hopeful or discouraged, so I closed the magazine, walked back to my room, and fell asleep as I listened to music.

※

I was in the lounge one morning when Dr. Tamargo debriefed me. That winter day in January, we sat facing each other across a cof-fee table. I think, "Without you, where would I be now?" I am grate-ful to this man and his skill. Later, I would learn more about his gifts. In August 1995, eight months after my surgery, he made the front page of the *Baltimore Sun*. "Suspended Animation used in Brain Surgery," the August 12 headline read. The accompanying photograph showed a three-and-a-half-month-old infant, Reginald Fitzgerald Jr., in his mother's arms. Doctors at Hopkins had lowered Reginald's temperature to sixty degrees, stopping his heart and slowing his circulation in a procedure called hypothermic circulatory arrest. Suspended animation, in popular terms. Stopping the heart gave Dr. Tamargo the time he needed to repair the large aneurysm in this patient, believed to be the youngest ever to undergo the procedure for that purpose. A few weeks later, the *Baltimore Afro-American* gave an update: the child's neurological exam revealed normal functioning. In November 1995, Dr. Tamargo made headlines again. This time he'd repaired an aneurysm in patient Shirley Glass, a York County, Pennsylvania, commissioner. As I read the newspaper accounts, I wondered if Dr. Tamargo could have saved my Aunt Vesta, who died from an aneurysm when I was a child.

Now, he tells me that my tumor was a meningioma, orange-sized, the third largest of its type, he'd believed, in the history of Hopkins Hospital. The tumor was benign. It had good margins, which meant that its edges contained the tissue; the tumor had not attached itself to many places on my brain. The tumor had grown on my left frontal lobe; that's why I had aphasia, muscle weakness, and other symptoms. I shouldn't be alarmed about my speech; many people who have brain surgery experience a temporary change in function. I would need plenty of rest.

I asked him about complications after surgery. I recalled choking and gasping for air. People ran to my side because my blood pressure dropped. They asked if I had a history of panic attacks. I thought how easy it would be for me to give up and just float away; I was tired. But I decided to live when I heard people telling me to hang on.

Dr. Tamargo said that my stay in the intensive care unit was uneventful; there were no emergencies. I surmised that I'd dreamed the blood pressure scene: too much medical drama on television perhaps? But reality is partly what you believe is "out there" and partly what you make of it. In that very first journal entry I'd written after surgery were these words:

I loved myself the moment my pressure dropped on the night of the operation. I didn't want to die. I am a child of God. God will take care of me.

※

On the day that Dr. Tamargo told me about the operation and the size of the tumor, I'd taken the news calmly. I think the shock hadn't worn off. I could not yet believe that on one day everybody, including me, thought I was OK, and a week later I had brain surgery. Two years later, at my annual MRI and consultation with Dr. Tamargo, I asked him to review the details of the operation. The surgery is called a craniotomy, and it involves cutting an opening through the skull, exposing the dura (the outermost covering of the central nervous system), and removing the tumor with an ultrasonic aspirator. The surgical team's work took hours, the better part of a day I will never forget even though I was unconscious during most of it.

※

Miraculous, everybody said. A few days after surgery, I was wheeled down to a room that looked like a small gym. There, physical therapists assessed me as I walked and carried out other ordinary motions. The therapists said my physical movement was normal. On rounds, I'd given the right responses to the requests the neurosurgical residents made to assess my functioning: smile (the right side of my mouth no longer drooped as it had before surgery); tell us what day it is; hold your arms straight out like you're holding a pizza. I could read, although I had trouble keeping track of the ideas. I could write one or two lines at a time.

But I was having difficulty recalling the names of things. I recall trips to the nurses' station when I was thirsty. I managed to get enough of a sentence out to indicate that I wanted a drink, and the nurses recited: Apple? Orange? Grape? Water? until I signaled my choice. The nurses assured me that the words would come and urged me to converse as much as possible. To help me understand how the tumor had affected me, one of the nurses gave me a postcard-sized picture with three views of the brain: the outside and top views of the left half (or hemisphere) and the inner view of the right half. The picture showed four color-coded lobes: salmon for the frontal, yellow for temporal, blue for parietal, and green for occipital. The cerebellum, the part next to the spinal cord, was white.

My tumor was on the left frontal lobe and had also pressed against the parietal lobe. The functions controlled by these two lobes were clearly marked. The parietal controlled sensations of touch, pressure, pain from the skin, and temperature. The frontal controlled concentration, planning, skills for solving problems, and motor control of voluntary muscles. The tumor's pressure on the left frontal lobe accounted for my preoperative smile that drooped on the right (the left side of the brain controls the right side of the body). The tumor's presence on the frontal lobe also accounted for my speech problems. I could not readily attribute the mood swings and irrational outbursts. A part of the brain called the limbic cortex controls emotional behavior, but the limbic cortex is buried deep in the brain.

※

The day my stitches were removed, I looked in the mirror and started crying and trembling. The surgical bandage had seemed almost like a fashionable, white turban; one of the residents said that sometimes patients feel a sense of security as long as the bandage is there. With it gone, the staples gleamed on the bald parts of my scalp. A little fringe of dull hair remained on the right edge; I looked like a clown.

I was discharged a week after surgery with two forms identifying the medications I needed and the conditions that would prompt a call to my physician. Barbara gathered the flowers and plants from my room, while I covered my head with the tam one of my friends had given me. While Barbara went ahead to get her van, I said good-bye to the nurses. I was grateful. All had shown exceptional skill, patience, and kindness. As the elevator carried me down to the lobby, I wondered what would happen when I got home, away from the nurses who had kept a twenty-four-hour watch on all of the patients on Meyer Nine.

The world outside the Hopkins hospital was cold, bright, sunny. As we drove back to my home in Columbia, I grasped the seat belts of Barbara's van so tightly that my nails left their imprint. In the real world, I could not take safety for granted. Anything could happen.

✵ Recovering Work

It is the first week of June 1995. I sit before a computer monitor in the rehab center. I promise I will treat myself to a manicure or a good mystery novel when I master this task. It requires me to remember a digit flashed for a second or two on the monitor, add the number to another digit that comes and goes just as quickly as the first, remember the sum, add it to another digit, and so on, all the while ignoring a digit, called a distracter, that flashes briefly in one of the corners of the monitor. I have to get a series of these correct before I can move to the next, more difficult level.

I have another two months to go before I end the rehab, to which I go three days a week for two hours each day—one hour for speech therapy and one hour for physical. The physical part is to relieve headaches and problems with my jaw and actually feels quite pleasant. The therapist is treating me with a method called craniosacral therapy, a relatively new process that uses touch to dispel the effects of trauma.

The speech part is work. I was expecting tasks that would speed up my speech or simple exercises to improve my memory. The diagnosis revealed that the fluent production of words was indeed one of my problems, but apparently I had sustained damage to brain functions regulating attention and concentration, which are needed for the efficient storage and recall of information. The treatment plan called for cognitive rehabilitation to improve my concentration and mental control, and language therapy to increase my retrieval of words. Without treatment, I would have difficulty remembering the names of students, memorizing and recalling details of research articles or new material in the textbooks I had ordered, lecturing without verbatim scripts, and participating in meetings.

I work hard to get things right, but I think of this part of my recovery as a job that I must do because I have no other options. I do not like learning skills that any fifth grader could do automatically: writing all the words that begin with a particular letter and doing so in what seems to be only seconds; writing the answers to questions after I've listened to a tape-recorded description (designed, I believe, to be complicated and dull); remembering the suit and number on playing cards. By the first week in July, I show mixed results: on one measure of fluency, I've gone from the 10th percentile to the 71st; on another, from the 15th to the 35th. My attention and concentration score is up, from the 29th percentile to the 73rd, but there is no change in my memory for words; I still score around the 35th percentile, which is low-average.

The rehab has become a daily reminder that the brain heals on its own schedule. There's no Prozac or lithium—no certain regimen that's been tried on large numbers of people and certified by the FDA. The side effects of brain surgery itself are sometimes unknown, only revealing themselves over time. Survivors are in limbo: we don't have a mental illness (like autism or schizophrenia), but our brains are different than before surgery. Presumably, we're better because of the repair, but we can also be worse.

Despite the fact that Dr. Tamargo gave me no milestones, I convinced myself that I would be back to normal in a few weeks—by Easter at the latest. After all, six months earlier and only one week after brain surgery, I arrived home from the hospital and stepped out of my friend Barbara's van slowly but unaided. From the sidewalk, I stepped up to the deck, walked slowly under the wisteria trellis, into my house, and straight into the arms of my mother, who said, "Let me hug my miracle child." I walked around the house. Everything was as I had left it—the photographs of my great-great-grandparents, Alex and Carrie, on the wall to the right of the front door; my collections of miniature houses arrayed in my bedroom, in a windowsill on the upstairs landing, on the kitchen counter; stacks and shelves of books in my study, the basement, and in all the bedrooms; quilts hanging on the curved stairwell, where I had fallen in September; some of the prints still stacked in corners waiting to be hung. I had moved into the house only six months before the operation.

Downstairs at the kitchen counter, Mom and Barbara figured out a schedule of medications. The two women, one in her seventies and the other barely forty-something, had known each other for less than an hour but were already a team. I was taking the six things I'd had in the hospital: Decadron, a steroid to reduce swelling in the brain; Dilantin, an antiseizure medicine; Zantac, to decrease stomach distress; Ativan, an antianxiety drug; and two hormones, estradiol and medroxyprogesterone, replacements for the natural hormones that decreased with menopause. The schedule was complicated by the gradual tapering required for the steroid, but I would stay on the Dilantin to control seizures; Dr. Tamargo had ordered it as a prophylactic. I was glad to have the medicine. What I feared most was a seizure like the one that sent me to the hospital—the loss of control over my mind and my body, followed by the loss of words and the loss of awareness.

Mom and Barbara wrote the times and doses for each of the medications, posted the schedule on the refrigerator, and left to pick up my prescriptions. I sat down in the kitchen. I was tired, not yet used to walking, talking, thinking what to say next, smiling, all the things people manage to do in ordinary interactions with family and friends. I was still in hospital mode—being done to, expected to respond to limited, benign commands and perfunctory requests.

Kali put a paper in my hands. She said something about tuition being due and how it was to be paid. I yelled, "Get away from me. Just go away," and started sobbing. Startled, Kali backed away. As soon as she heard Mom and Barbara's footsteps on the porch, she ran to the front door, explaining how she didn't mean to upset me. They said all the best things: I might have looked OK, but I was still recovering; I needed to take a dose of medicine; I needed to get to bed; I'd only been home an hour, and I was exhausted by the trip from the hospital.

The confrontation over tuition left me with the certainty that, miracle or not, the world hadn't stopped because I had had brain surgery. I was still a mother, a tenured professor, a researcher. The bills came in, right on schedule. A student called with a request that I reread her final paper; she hoped for a higher grade. An officer from the National Science Foundation called to ask if I would serve on a panel to review proposals. The vice president of a university asked me to apply for a position in the education department. A colleague gently insisted that I honor a commitment to write a chapter for her forthcoming book.

Dr. Tamargo said I would be able to work from home within weeks. But teaching is a complex task, he told me, and he advised me not to return to the classroom until the following semester. Fortunately, my colleagues had already arranged to cover my classes. I could do the rest of my work—preparing lectures, writing, advising students, compiling technical reports for Hopkins—with the aid of a home computer and fax. I would still have an income. I had excellent health insurance; except for copayments, the tens of thousands of dollars in hospital bills and physicians fees would be covered. And, more important than anything else, I had the love and support of family, friends, and colleagues.

※

I got through February, the first month after surgery, with the kind of discipline that I'd learned in the home of two public school teachers. My parents' weekdays had had little flexibility. In addition to getting three of their own children up, fed, and dressed, they were responsible for getting their students through days marked by scheduled lessons, lunchtimes, after-school conferences and activities. On weekends, my parents had a different routine. Saturday mornings we cleaned house; each of us had a set of chores. Afternoons were for enrichment—going to the library, piano lessons, dance lessons. Sundays we went to Sunday school and church, and afterward, to my grandmother's house for dinner.

My routine revolved around pills and meals. I didn't have to think about it; my mother kept time, waking at 5 A.M. to give me a snack and medication; dozing until 7, when she woke me for breakfast and more medication; sitting with me in my study as I read a little, tried to write. She made lunch around noon and told me to rest afterward. In the afternoons, she and I chatted with the colleague who'd volunteered that day to bring us a home-cooked dinner. Thanks to my Hopkins colleagues, we had a month of treats, from crabmeat quiche to home-baked rolls and ratatouille.

My mother and I grew closer, perhaps because I saw how she must have cared for me when I was a young child. I think she saw the little girl in me who always insisted, I can do this myself, and watched for the times when I faltered. I bathed and dressed myself from the first day I returned from the hospital, but I didn't like to look in the mirror; the thought of seeing and touching my stitches frightened and dismayed me. My mother stepped in; my stitches had to be cleaned each day to prevent infection. Mom would dip a swab in peroxide and gently wipe the half-U that looked like bird footprints in a field of snow. "One wants a Teller in times like this," wrote the poet Gwendolyn Brooks. Mom was my Teller, reassuring me, "Be patient, time brings all good things," and, I hoped, "(and cool / Strong balm to calm the burning at the brain?)."

In the mornings when I was alert, I did the tasks that came from the outside world. With my mother's help, I wrote checks. I read the student's paper and wrote a critique; it took three days to write one page. I started an outline for the chapter my colleague wanted. I covered my baldness with one of those paper bonnets that hospital and food workers wear and visited with friends who stopped by. There were times when I would speak only to pause mid-sentence with a space for where a word should have gone. Strangely, I had no trouble with curses. One evening, my mother, Barbara, and other friends were sitting at the kitchen table. The conversation was light. Someone said something about a person I didn't particularly like anymore, and I said something like, "There's a real asshole," and other comments with more than a few expletives, perfectly timed and spoken. It was quiet for a second as everyone looked at my mother, who didn't seem shocked at all. We laughed.

On weekends my daughters would join my mom and me, and I tried to follow their conversations. Kali and Alana were delighted to get to know their grandmother better, and the three of them talked about everything from courses the girls were taking to the amazing diversity—racial and career-wise—of my friends. I listened to the news and repeated to myself what I could remember. I watched the "Trial of the Century" and tried to summarize the proceedings for my mother. I gained weight; steroids give you an outrageous appetite. I walked a little to regain my physical strength, first to the mailbox in the courtyard, careful to avoid the four-year-old who waved a tree limb that had fallen during a storm (I was afraid my head would crack at the surgical fault line), then in late February with Mom and Marcia, my neighbor, through the mall, avoiding mirrors that showed another residue of the steroids—the beginnings of hair everywhere but on my head.

I had started writing in my journal again on February 5, with one

sentence: *"I just got over brain surgery."* On the tenth, I tried to write
a poem:

Crazy visitation, a friend calls
The tumor
Brainless,
from my brain
not of it.

Meningioma, surgeons call
The tumor:
Useless,
for removal only.

Sleeping spirit, I call
The tumor:
Tissue nourished on nightmares
repository of anger.

My symptoms cried and seized,
Cut it out! And surgeons did,
making space for
spirits of many names:
Grateful, graceful,
Exuberant,
Awake.

I call them!

But I had difficulty finding the right words, the right rhythm; my journal shows that I tried for about two weeks to complete the poem: phrases were crossed-out, I had many false starts, and it seems that my memory failed me when I'd written two or three letters where there should have been a word. Although I sent the draft to my writers' group, I never revised the poem to my satisfaction.

As the weeks went by, I could work for longer periods, but I still felt fatigued and sluggish. I wrote in my journal: "peaks and valleys, highs and lows." Although the drugs slowed my thoughts and I tired easily and felt like Humpty-Dumpty, I thought I was making progress in speech, which I read as the main sign that my brain itself was healing. But one night, early in February, I awakened during the night with a temperature of more than one hundred degrees; it remained so for twenty-four hours. I called Dr. Tamargo, who suspected an allergic reaction to the antiseizure medication. He changed me to another medicine, carbamazepine (Tegretol), and asked me to come in at mid-month for a check on the drug level in my blood.

Waiting in the lobby of the outpatient clinic for my mother and the friend who had driven us to the appointment, I saw people who were wheeled in and out of the building and those who walked with a swaying gait. Some talked too slowly or spoke with no pauses, in monotones; some did not speak at all. I saw those whose eyes wandered, gently refusing to focus. And there were those whose hair had been shorn, sometimes in odd ways, like mine was under the green wool tam that a friend had given me a few days before the operation. "It's cold out," she'd said. "You'll need something to protect your head when you leave the hospital."

I used to look away from people like the ones in the clinic, but I could no longer avert my gaze. I'd crossed over and joined those whose primary work was recovery. That morning, I asked Dr. Tamargo to tell me what to do. Is there a way to speed up the process? He reminded me that I had had a very serious operation that lasted more than six hours. I needed time to heal, but I should do anything I could to stimulate my brain and keep my spirits high. What caused this? I asked. Was it stress, the Vivactyl and lithium I'd taken for depression? No, he'd said, the tumor probably had been growing right along with you. I asked are there any books I can read, any information? He gave me one title, *Death Be Not Proud,* and suggested that I contact the American Brain Tumor Association. He reminded me that much remains to be discovered about the connection between mind and body, and we talked about my depression, which seemed to have evaporated. He cautioned me to wait and see. Sometimes, he said, patients are happy simply because they are alive.

I was confident that Dr. Tamargo would be one of my partners in my physical healing, and Maureen, my psychotherapist, would help me sort out the emotional rubble left in the wake of the divorce, the job change, and the tumor. Some things I would have to do for myself: get up every day, gracefully accept help for things that I had so successfully accomplished on my own before surgery, and find the will, the spirit, and the patience to regain my intellectual power and my confidence. In my journal, I described my intensified efforts to recover as *"a 2000 piece puzzle that I could never put together under any circumstances."*

I renewed my efforts by asking: what did I have left after the double loss of a partner and my health? What had others who had gone before me retrieved from their derailed lives? I wanted to know about real people who had undergone brain surgery. How had they handled the news that someone had to cut a hole in the scalp and peel it back, drill holes in their skull, saw away the bone using the holes as endpoints, remove the skull parts and put them aside, and suck or cut away the diseased tissue in the brain?

For inspiration, I read the book that Dr. Tamargo had recommended; the teenage son of the journalist who wrote the book died of his brain tumor. One of my neighbors brought a copy of *Grace and Grit*, the story of a woman who had breast cancer followed by cancer of the brain. The heroes in both of these books learned to live one breath at a time. *A Whole New Life*, a memoir by Reynolds Price, was published that spring. Price became a paraplegic in his fifties; a large tumor had invaded his spine. His was a slow and painful recovery: years passed as he underwent rehabilitation, chemotherapy, radiation, and varied remedies for pain. The book soon became my constant companion, both for the beauty of his writing and the insights on suffering, disability, and divine grace.

I remembered that Quincy Jones had had a brain operation. I read his biography and discovered that he'd had not one but two operations to repair a brain aneurysm. And I recalled the story of Tammi Terrell, who collapsed onstage in the arms of Marvin Gaye, when they were performing a duet. I bought *Every Great Motown Hit of Marvin*

Gaye and soothed myself with the sounds of "you're all I need to get by."

One day I received in the mail an article on social support from Joe Pleck, the colleague who was my coauthor for a book chapter on resilience and African American adolescents. In the margins Joe had written, "I care about you." Joe and I had reviewed many studies that revealed that despite adversity, many black teens had done well in school and in their relationships with others. They, like adults and children in different racial and economic groups, overcame hard times with a combination of help from others and personal qualities like spirituality and religious faith, persistence, and a sense of competence.

Research tells us that multiple forms of support from others are necessary to reduce mental health problems that can occur after the negative and uncontrollable stress of medical illness. Assets in the form of good medical insurance and aspects of work that I could carry out from home were important, but without the vigorous response of my family, friends, and colleagues, I could not have faced the isolation and despair of a life-threatening illness. While I was in the hospital, they provided emotional support by giving messages of love and caring. After I left the hospital, my network responded with love and instrumental support such as meals, names of competent and trusted medical professionals, and transportation while I could not drive.[1]

I had the social support, and I could rebuild the personal, if need be. I interpreted Joe's note as "Saundra, you know about this resilience stuff. You know what to do."

But beneath the calm determination to get better, my anger was growing, fueled in part by suggestions from friends.

"You should get yourself a good lawyer," one friend, a psychologist, said to me in late February, as my mother and I sat at her table for dinner. Her husband, also a psychologist, showed me some lines in a neuropsychology text. "See," he said, "the three major symptoms of a brain tumor are aphasia, muscle weakness, and depression. You had all three when you went to the emergency room, and no one bothered to check your head."

Although a good many friends hinted that I should sue, I was ambivalent. When you're fresh from being under the knife, you feel relief, not desire for retribution. And I was still smarting from the last legal hassle, my divorce. My anger came out through the question "Why me?"

Some say that it is a waste of time to ask. I didn't say the words out loud so that others could hear, but surreptitiously in my own mind, where I had difficulty hearing it myself. Mom and I went to the bookstore, and I looked for Rabbi Kushner's book *When Bad Things Happen to Good People*, because I'd always said I would read it, but now I had a very good excuse to do so. The book helped, assuring me that I hadn't done anything to deserve this on a moral level, that God hadn't kept score and made me an understudy for Job.

At the end of February my mother returned to Atlanta, where my father was recuperating from glaucoma surgery he'd had the week before mine. After she left, I lay idle.

My friends still called and asked if I needed anything; I had the occasional visitor who dropped by with flowers or food. My neighbors had the keys to my house and assured me that I could call on them in emergencies or if I wanted company. My daughters came home on weekends when they didn't have dorm duties; both had jobs as resident advisors. Without my mother's constant presence; the predictable, daily coming and going of daughters and friends; and the regimen of drugs, I was on my own. I followed the schedule that my mother and I had established. The crisis was over.

※

Shocked and depleted, for almost three weeks I did very little. I performed my daily tasks by rote, grateful for the respite of sleep. I faked a cheery tone when people called, or said I was drowsy when I didn't feel like talking. I stared out of my window for hours listening to Mozart's *Requiem* or Coltrane's *A Love Supreme*. Sometimes I watched old movies and reruns of everything.

When you've lost your mind—or had it taken temporarily in surgery, knocked out so you don't think for hours—it comes back in little pieces. One night I awoke suddenly, smiling with the memory of a dream of blue skies, green meadows, brown people in yellow and red clothes. I believe it was the first dream I'd had in color for months. Avoiding the scarred, tender area on the left side of my head, I propped myself on three pillows and gazed each day at a large tree framed by the glass door opposite my bed. Until the buds opened, I followed the daily passage of a family of squirrels who lived near the top. I saw the flashy reds of cardinals and wanted to write a poem about them, but couldn't find the words. I saw how rain responds to changes in the wind, light, temperature. By myself for much of the time, without the distraction of cheerful others, I became aware of each change, no matter how minor, in my energy and my moods, the twinges of body parts, the surges of blood, the sounds and rhythms of my breath and heart, the workings of my mind. I was afraid something else

Recovering Work   103

would surprise me—a thief in the night, another seizure, perhaps a stroke or a bolt of lightning. I was the watcher, the observant guard, perhaps resetting a timer in some hidden part of me to the beat of nature; the professional clock that for twenty years had measured the doer by the length of my resume was still.

My daughters, themselves fatigued by the demands of school, part-time jobs, and checking in on me, were appalled by the replacement of their capable, upbeat mother with one who was passive, listless, and uncertain. "Mom, get over it," Alana said one day when she caught me in tears. "You don't act like a survivor. You should be happy."

Kali agreed. "We want our mother back," she said.

How does the brain cleanse its own wounds? Relearn the signals to balance the body as it walks through the forest? Reset the synchronous inner rhythms of the systems that emanate from the fragile coiled mass, guarded from human eyes by skull and skin? Scientists can't observe the workings of the human brain as it heals. Certainly my daughters could not, nor could I. On the outside, I looked fine.

Three years later, when they were twenty-three and told their own versions of this episode, my daughters explained their fears. Alana had no vision of what I would become; she knew only that she did not want me to regress to the fatigued and weak shell I was during the two years before the diagnosis. She wanted me to take advantage of a more relaxed pace than I'd had in those years when I was ill but didn't know why and worked late and on weekends anyway. Kali's concern was different. She recognized my competitive streak. I constantly measured the milestones of my life—the Ph.D., the birth of the children, the houses—against the highest standards I could find.

✴

Nights were bad. I longed for someone—a partner, a companion, to rub my back or hold me or maybe just share the events of the days. But I remembered that I was never alone. Sometimes I'd stare at the images of my family members, especially the photograph of Carrie and Alex in the cotton field. My racial heritage became an unexpected source of strength, perhaps because it took me out of myself, connecting my personal efforts to regain my competence to community needs and legacies of struggle. Mary Helen Washington, writing about the message in black women's writings, reminds us that "we cannot be committed simply to ourselves."

I'd say a prayer or think of Christ on the cross, and I thought about my angel and the presence that assured me: *everything is all right*. The loneliness would vanish and in its place were feelings of relief that I could focus on getting myself well instead of being concerned about the sadness, anger, or disgust that my bald head, my weight, or my halting speech might have stirred in someone who would be with me. My lifelong commitment to seeking meaning through religious faith provided me with an ideology that enabled me to see suffering and struggle as part of life. The images I had of Christ on the cross foreshadowed the possibilities for renewal and psychological wholeness after physical disaster. My faith linked me to a community of believers who prayed for my life when I could not pray for myself, but my sense of a higher power present in my life made it easier for me to be in solitude, finding solace through meditation and reading, especially the writings of others whose narratives of illness were couched in spiritual terms.

And I had the tumor, more palpable in the aftermath of its removal than it ever was when no one knew it was there.

※

In mid-March, my colleague Gary drove me to appointments at the Hopkins clinic. The initial one was for my first MRI since the operation. Then I'd been unfazed, in a drug-induced haze; the procedure seemed innocuous. Now, my heart raced, and I shivered when I saw the apparatus—a gleaming white capsule into which the patient slides prone on a narrow slab. The technician gave me earphones through which I could listen to music, and I lay with a light blanket on my body (the room was chilly). The slab began rolling into the cylinder. "Keep your head perfectly still," the technician said, "or else we might have to repeat the scan. Try not to swallow until a break in the scan." I was inside the capsule for about twenty-five minutes; the technician slid me back out and injected a dye into my right arm and slid me back inside for another twenty minutes. When the machine was on and I was in the capsule, I heard knocking sounds that completely drowned out the music. I wanted desperately to go to the bathroom, to yell, "Get me out," and to gulp down excess saliva, all at the same time. I repeated the Twenty-third Psalm the whole time, and sneaked a swallow.

About an hour after the MRI, I saw Dr. Tamargo, who said the preliminary results of the scan showed a large area of blood deposits on the left side where the tumor had been. He assured me that I needn't worry about them; they were part of the healing process. He gave me the go-ahead to work longer hours at home and gradually resume as much of a normal life as possible, and he wrote a prescription for speech therapy. A therapist had evaluated me soon after I was discharged from the hospital and found some deficits that weren't apparent to me.

After the appointments, Gary and I had lunch with another friend, John Holland, at a favorite Thai restaurant near the Hopkins campus. We talked about professional affairs. Gary and John were revising a dictionary of careers based on John's psychological instrument that helps determine which careers fit your personality. We didn't talk about the tumor, and I didn't have to say much. These two friends have a droll wit, and I laughed a lot, especially when they teased that I looked like a character from Winnie the Pooh in the floppy hat I wore to hide the fuzz growing around my scar.

After Gary dropped me at home, I sat in my living room, idly turning the pages of one of my books on African American art and photography. Usually, the books are neatly stacked in two piles, and large hardbound volumes of work by my favorite artist, Romare Bearden, anchor both. I was tired, but I smiled as I recalled an exchange in the clinic that morning. I was standing in the registration line when a noticeably younger man said, "Hi. You're single?" To which I replied, "Why do you ask?" "Because you're so beautiful and well-spoken."

Now, I can recognize a line when I hear one, but it had been months since I had the pleasure of a casual flirtation. Sexual feelings of even the mildest sort were, it seemed, a thing of the past. "I'm just getting over a brain operation," I said, pointing to my hat. "I used to have poor judgment in men, but maybe the operation took that away." We both laughed, and that was that.

✤

I began to dread teaching classes after a day in March when a colleague drove me to the office to gather the books I would use in the fall, copies of journal articles, and my mail. Two brown envelopes with white labels were among the catalogs, notices, and requests for this and that. They contained student evaluations from the previous fall, when I hadn't realized how ill I was. I opened them and felt hot and dizzy. If ever I felt replaceable, it was when I read my students' comments. A small, really minuscule, proportion was complimentary, and overall, I got high ratings for my knowledge. But on other categories the students were merciless. One of them wrote, "She was horrible, horrible." I felt that way as I read through the evaluations and wondered if my memory lapses, slurred speech, and equilibrium problems had contributed to students' stereotypes about the competence of black professors. Despite the warm greetings from my colleagues and their wishes for my health, I left the office feeling like a fraud. I was beginning to doubt the progress that I'd made. Where was my old energy? My old ability to lecture without extensive notes? My old spontaneity in discussions? My ability to write and read for hours at a time? Lost, it seemed in the blood-lined crater that Dr. Tamargo had described.

On the way home, my colleague and I talked about how the tumor might have created my unconfident and often bizarre behavior before the operation. In the weeks I had been recuperating, more incidents than I cared to remember came back to me. One of them concerned the third course I'd added to my schedule during my first semester at UM. On the evening I lectured, I did the last things you want to do in front of a group of teachers: dropped my notes, flubbed my sentences, spoke in a soft monotone, blanked out completely when the students engaged in a lively conversation about the topic. One student wrote feedback that went something like, "She needs to enroll in a Toastmasters' course."

At other times, I had done things that were just plain out of character for me, and I recalled them with embarrassment. In a meeting between my evaluation team and the people who funded us, I blurted out something mean about a man from my past, a person who had nothing to do with the agenda. I left rude phone mail messages for scholars who wanted to meet with me. I churned the same thoughts in the same ways because I could not think of anything new. At conferences and meetings, I gave irrelevant answers to simple questions. I addressed another scholar by a popular rap singer's name, and repeated that name every time I had to say something to her.

※

In "A Matter of Identity," an essay from *The Man Who Mistook His Wife for a Hat*, the neurologist Oliver Sacks tells the true tale of Mr. Thompson, a Korsakov's patient. Korsakov's syndrome is a severe impairment of memory; neural pathways are damaged in ways that interfere with memory of recent events. Mr. Thompson could recall impressions from his childhood and adolescence, but since the disease began (a result of alcoholism), he had no sense of himself from day to day, minute to minute. He continually improvised, assuming different identities and the activities of whomever he decided momentarily to be: now a delicatessen owner, then a reverend. Sacks wrote, "We have, each of us, a life-story, an inner narrative—whose continuity, whose sense is our lives. It might be said that each of us constructs and lives, a 'narrative,' and that this narrative is us, our identities."[2] Deprived of the inner narrative, Mr. Thompson could not hold on to his identity.

I'd not had as permanent a disruption of identity as Mr. Thompson, but the tumor had undermined my motivation, confidence, and desire to be a teacher, an identity toward which many episodes of my life seemed to point. In my earliest memories, I am teaching. My classroom was in the backyard of our house on DeSoto Street in Atlanta. The room was really a shed that ran the length of the garage to which it was attached. It had windows, a door, and a sloping roof and served at various times as a doghouse, a tool shed, and a playhouse. My pupils were my brother and sister, any cousins who happened to be visiting (my family, my uncle's family, and my grandparents shared a large house), and the children in the neighborhood. What I taught was anything that happened to be interesting to me on a given day—how to spell, Greek architecture, reading. In my high school yearbook, a photographer caught me in front of a blackboard, glasses in hand, explaining a science project called "The Solar House." Architecture was, and remains, another passion.

At midlife, I'd seemed to be putting it all together with the faculty appointment at Maryland. Now, I wanted to hide behind a computer terminal and never have to communicate with groups of people again. I toyed with the idea of a research job in the South to be near my relatives, but the prospect of putting myself back in the job market was too frightening to consider. So was moving from our house, which I was beginning to love. And most of all, being a long distance from my daughters.

In April my friend Fran came from Detroit to visit me for a week, along with her grandson Chance, her daughter Myla, and one of Myla's friends. Fran is an elegant, fashionable woman, and has been so since we first met as librarians in Howard University's Moorland-Spingarn collection, which houses materials on the African diaspora. Our bonds became stronger as we went through our divorces, became single mothers raising daughters, attended graduate school to earn our doctorates, and remarried, in Fran's case, quite happily. With her help, I began to do things that I needed to do to regain my stamina and confidence. For exercise, we walked to the park in my neighborhood. Myla, a vegetarian, cooked stir-frys and pasta while Fran and I talked and sipped herbal tea. Before she returned to Detroit, she said, "Buzz cuts and big earrings are in fashion. Get rid of that floppy hat."

Mother's Day, 1995. Money was very tight, and I hadn't wanted Alana and Kali to buy presents, so they wrote a note.

Dear Mom,

On this Mother's Day, Kali and I decided to reflect upon our experience with you this year. We think we never realized what you meant until the night you went into the hospital.

Alana: The thought of a woman who gave me wisdom with all of our personal development chats, the person who told me "It's all about what you want," the mom who always strove to support my ever changing majors and far flung dreams not being a part of my life made me crazy with fear and gave me a sense of hopelessness. But for some reason, even in the darkness of the moment, I knew you would survive.

Kali: During your illness, all I could think about was your hands. When I was a child, those hands personified elegance and beauty. Mom, without you, I would not have, for a lack of a better word, culture, that inexpressible need for what is good and beautiful in this world.

We didn't want conclusions because there is no conclusion to our never-ending love.

I folded the note, written on creamy paper with lacy etching, and placed it in the pocket of the notebook with my daily calendar. The note would be my reminder that my children looked to me for some of what they needed in this life: support, wisdom, love, and the ability to see the beauty in themselves and in the world. Now, with this illness, I could show them something more: a kind of graceful vulnerability, the attitude that says *weakened, yes; victim, no.*

I did what I had to do to return to the world beyond my front door. After two months of denial that I needed speech therapy, I called a rehabilitation center for an intake evaluation and signed on for treatment. I resumed my weekly trips to Maureen for counseling and psychotherapy. I began and ended my days with prayer and practiced what I later learned was a form of walking meditation, which consists of simply paying attention to each step and nothing else. I talked regularly to my parents, my sister, Barbara, Fran, and others who wanted the best for me. I submitted a formal application to participate in an interdisciplinary research seminar, "Representations and

Meanings of Black Women's Work," at UM. In my letter of application to Black Women and Work, as the project came to be known, I wrote: "The seminar would be an opportunity for me to focus on ways that mothers model work-related resilience and how sons and daughters construct meaning using the successful adaptation of their mothers as guides."

I continued to read articles and books for my lectures, noting ideas for discussions. In one of my classes, I planned to present information on plasticity, the organism's capacity to adapt to diverse conditions. I found a perfect example to illustrate the point while leafing through a sourcebook of popular and technical literature on human development. A reprint from *Life* magazine, the article was "Building a Better Brain," and it explained that scientists had once thought that brain circuits changed little beyond adolescence. Research tells us that this view is outmoded. Neurons, the cells in the brain, can grow new dendrites, the appendages at one end of the cell. To my eyes, dendrites resemble the fragile roots that grow from a philodendron stem immersed in water. Dendrites can be stimulated to branch by exercises, such as crossword puzzles, that challenge the mind. The more branches, the more connections between brain cells. The more connections, the faster the mind works and the more tasks it can perform. This information about neuroplasticity, the ways in which the brain can repair itself, was in line with what Dr. Tamargo had told me.

In addition to reading for work, I found other ways to strengthen my mind. I filled my journals with lessons gleaned from books I read and movies I watched. I reflected on the film *Searching for Bobby Fisher*: "*Too much pressure (external or internal) ruins the joy of the game. Take time out for living other things. Be a decent person. Find the other guy a way out."* One day, I wrote, *"I spent the morning reading A* Path with Heart: A Guide Through the Perils and Promises of Spiritual Life, *trying to make some sense out of my doubt, my wanting. After I read the section on the dark night of the soul, I knew that I've gone through it and known the sense of resting, the sense of peace."*

As I read, I monitored my energy, the tiredness of my eyes, the digression of my thoughts, and my wandering attention. Still, I had to reread information and make copious notes before I could remember material. I went through the same procedure as I was writing the chapter my colleague had demanded, which was about resiliency in adolescents. On this project, I discovered the common aspects in three theories. It took me longer to grasp the essential notion, and I wondered whether or not the Tegretol slowed my thought. But, I figured, that one "aha" was a sign that more would follow. In my journal I wrote notes for enlivening class discussions, notes on interesting things I encountered in my reading, notes for the kind of relationship I wanted with students. I see now that I minimized the role that my speech, my voice, would take: *"teaching/listener; teaching/listening, telling/hearing,"* I wrote.

�֍

It is mid-August 1995, and I sit at a desk, my lecture notes stacked neatly in front of me. The speech therapist adjusts the video camera. "Ready?" she says, and steps away from the tripod. I have rehearsed the notes many times at home before today's taping, but I still stumble over the opening lines. This is just the first of several sessions, practice to get me ready for the real thing, my first class since the surgery.

We tape for twenty minutes or so and then review the tape. A few seconds in, the therapist stops the tape. Although Dr. Tamargo took me off the Tegretol a few days ago, I speak slowly and softly. I still feel a dull ache when I open my mouth wide enough to project my voice. The therapist suggests that I order a hand-held microphone; she tells me that people often use them after head surgery. They give you something to hold on to. She pushes the play button, stops the tape, critiques my performance.

It was only the second image I'd seen of myself since the surgery. The first had been a Polaroid picture snapped in the shadows at a table in our favorite restaurant; the occasion was a special one, Alana and Kali's twentieth birthday on July 1. The girls, one on either side of me, are grinning. Kali has one arm around my shoulder; Alana leans against me. My lips are parted as if I fear getting too happy, being too happy. As if another bad surprise looms ahead.

I stare at the video image trying to match the person on the tape with the me in my mind. The tape shows my sluglike moves; I weigh 142 pounds, twenty-five of them gained since I left the hospital. I cannot keep a steady gaze. My eyes are hooded and dull.

The image I want to be was captured ten, maybe eleven, years earlier, and comes from my favorite photograph. I am in Las Vegas at a conference. I am smiling, divorced after fourteen years, and in the midst of my first romance; my eyes sparkle, my skin glows. My hair is full and shiny and touches my shoulders. I stand at ease and look directly into the camera. I am carefree for once, and I have a list of things I want to accomplish in the future: dance and music lessons for the girls, a job in academe, a novel, a new house.

Now my hair is still cut in a very short Afro; it has not grown at the half-inch per month that the nurses said it would. People have remarked often that the hairdo is stunning; I hate the look and have missed my hair the way, perhaps, amputees miss their limbs. My vain complaints prompted Alana to ask me, "Mom, which would you rather have? Your hair or your life?"

The life, of course. But the mantra of the normal mind is "more"— more joy, more love, more knowledge, more range of motion. More hair. Right now, I want the confident person I was in that moment in Las Vegas, before the pills for depression, the second marriage and divorce, the tumor.

But the present life is what I see on the video, and I have been going on with that life for months. I leave the rehab center and go for a walk. By now, my physical stamina has improved so much that I can make a complete circuit—about a mile and a half—around the small lake in the park. When I get home, I see the wisteria, twisted across the trellis that shelters my front porch. I remembered the fragrant white blossoms, which bloomed the past May. A haiku comes to me spontaneously:

Whispering
the white wisteria send a scented message:
Home now.

Later that day I work on some reports, go to my writers' group, and record in my journal, *"a very good day."*

The next morning, my speech therapist hugs me when I repeat the haiku for her. The fluent production of words has been one of our goals. When the treatment program ends on August 29, I score in the 98th percentile on a measure of word fluency. Although my verbal memory is average, around the 75th percentile, it, too, is up from the low-average range. My attention and concentration, which showed a mild deficit when I first entered speech therapy, is now in the high-average category. I think, "This is great, I'm on a roll." It seems as if the rehab and all the other things I tried to do to improve my brain are having a positive effect. The day before classes begin, I write, "We are here to transcend the struggle."

✸ Mourning into Dancing

It is October 1998, and I sit in the noisy dining room in the University of Maryland's student union building. "Doc Nettles, mind if I sit here?" I look up from the essay I am grading. Gary, a.k.a. "Thunder," is already sliding in the bench across the table from me. "Sure," I say. "What's up?" We chat about his assignment and one of the topics we'd discussed that day in class. The conversation shifts to another topic: how Gary reacted when he was diagnosed with lymphatic cancer. He told me about the cancer the first day of class and that sometimes he would have to miss classes when he had treatments.

"I used to be a shit," Gary says. "You wouldn't have liked me. I was the kind of person who put other people down, made fun of them." He leans on the table, looks me right in the eye, pulls the lid of his baseball cap over his thinning hairline. "This thing changed my life. You've been there. You know." I nod and say, "I used to be a star. People said that I had great potential." I check my watch, embarrassed. I am not used to disclosing feelings to students.

"I've got to run to class. I enjoyed our little chat," I say and stand up, but Gary has more to say.

"Dr. Nettles, you went through that brain operation and you've lived to tell about it. You're still a star."

We go in opposite directions. I am halfway across the dining room when someone yells, "Hey Doc!" I turn and see Gary walking rapidly toward me. "Here's something that I just made up: S.T.A.R. It means 'Start Thinking and Acting Resilient.'"

"I like it," I say, smiling. "See you in class on Thursday."

I walk outside. Maryland is in the midst of a months-long drought; the leaves on the mature trees that dot the campus are dry and golden. It is warm today, and students are in jeans and T-shirts.

I think about Gary and what he said to me. I feel that I do well these days. I am enjoying my classes for the first time since I came to UM, but I still appreciate the reminders of how precious each day is.

※

Such a conversation would never have occurred three years ago, when I returned to the classroom in fall 1995. I would like to say that my reentry was as smooth as a routine landing of a spacecraft, but I was anxious, and it showed. My department ordered a microphone for me, but it wouldn't arrive for weeks, so I strained to project my voice in my first class, a large graduate course with more than twenty students. The class met from four until seven o'clock; I had been in my office most of the day and was weary by the time class began. Some of the old terror from my nightmarish first semester worked its way from my heart outward to all my limbs. I soon had rings of perspira tion on my linen jacket and little drops lined up around my hairline. All my practice with paying attention only to what I had to do right now deserted me, and my mind flipped a playback switch. As in the days before the tumor was diagnosed, I found myself stuttering, trying to get the words out, my heart booming in double time, my balance sensors set to sway, drag right leg.

The students were still, waiting for me to begin. I glanced at the first woman in the front row. She smiled and introduced herself. "I'm Cindy," she said. Later, she would be the first doctoral student assigned to me. Then, I think Cindy's smile brought me back. I remembered that I could apply the mnemonic devices I learned during rehab to recall my students' names, but I found it difficult to transfer the skills that I'd practiced in isolation to a classroom with twenty-three unfamiliar faces. I explained the syllabus, gave an introductory talk about the nature of social development, and invited the class to join the discussion. I was distracted by my own thoughts: had they noticed that I was slightly off? I'd felt the lag between my thoughts and my words. I recalled the days when my brainwork was silent, below my ability to detect. Finally, I decided to confess: "I'm recovering from brain surgery, so please bear with me if my words come out slowly at times, or sound scrambled." I looked for the faces expressing disdain—"She has her nerve, trying to get sympathy"—or doubt—"Is she brain damaged?" It surprised me when my students were curious instead. "Did you have headaches?" was the first question in both of my classes. "When did you first find out? Was your tumor benign or malignant? Are you OK now?"

At the end of the first week of classes, I returned to another part of the scholarly world, the discussions among peers about ideas and events. I was apprehensive about whether I could still function in the sometimes intense give-and-take, but I had already committed myself to participate in the Black Women and Work seminar, the multidisciplinary group of eighteen professors at Maryland and other campuses in the Washington, D.C., area. We met for a two-day retreat at a conference center in the Virginia countryside, and during the first session, I said to one of the scholars, "I can't think this way, use this type of language." More than a decade had passed since I'd had the time or brainpower to train a critical eye on questions such as, what is reality and how can we know it? An intellectual debate was going on between scholars who say we can apprehend reality and those who say human beings construct it. I awakened from a tumorous sleep to confront an academic world in which people spoke of chaos theory and the deconstruction of texts. My comment led to a discussion of how we could juggle the diverse interests of the various disciplines we represented: law, literary criticism, history, anthropology, sociology, and psychology.

By the end of the second day when we posed for a group picture, I found myself laughing and joking with the rest of the participants as we lined up. I was relieved. I had no trouble following the logic of the discussions, and I had forgotten myself as we engaged in lively conversation and respectful debate. I sensed the beginning of a very special way of connecting our diverse styles and scholarly disciplines, and I was eager to meet again. I felt balanced for the first time in months; my brain, my spirit, my body were working in sync. The retreat gave me the courage to say yes at the first faculty meeting of the semester when the chair called for a volunteer to present a research talk to our department.

In the middle of that September, Dr. Tamargo and I chatted about my progress when I visited the Johns Hopkins outpatient clinic for an MRI and consultation. My brain had repaired itself well enough to perform the basic tasks that before had eluded me. I could remember phone numbers and figure out the amount of tips to leave at restaurants. My body seemed to be awakening from the anesthetic slumber: as long as I kept a steady flow of food to my brain, I could stay up longer, walk farther and faster. My emotions were regular, appropriate, not morphing wildly.

I told Dr. Tamargo about my classes, which were going about as well as could be expected, given that when my symptoms intensified, during the fall of 1994, I gave little sustained thought to the fact that I was in a new job. I didn't share with him some unsettling questions that came up the minute I'd set foot on campus. One concern was whether I would be able to put aside my queasiness when I faced white students. When I'd taught years before, most of my students were African Americans, and I could interpret the nonverbal signs signaling that something I had said was misunderstood or hadn't been heard at all. Despite having presented several papers at scientific meetings attended primarily by whites, I'd never felt attuned to those audiences. Although my colleagues at Hopkins and Maryland were white, they were known, and in some cases, beloved friends. I attributed my lingering uneasiness to the fact that until I was twenty and graduated from Howard University, I had lived in a segregated world. I was also aware that I didn't fit the usual image of a professor at a major university. With about 5 percent of the faculty being African Americans, Maryland had a larger proportion than other comparable universities. Even though other black people were around, I'd been one of less than a handful in some of my classes, and the only one in others.

The other question was one for which Dr. Tamargo had already given a wait-and-see answer. Would I regain the intellectual power and energy that I displayed years before the tumor was diagnosed? Now that I had mastered basics like concentrating and recalling spoken and written words, I wanted to think quickly on a higher order. Many days I heard my thoughts clunking like the central processing unit of one of those early personal computers. My ability to think abstractly—a necessity for my work—was improving by what psychologists call "jnd's," or just noticeable differences. These are changes in perception so subtle, so slight, that you can miss them if you don't pay attention. So slowly came the changes that I wondered if my colleagues would think I was dead weight, no longer able to keep apace of demands. I'd believed myself to be resilient and strong; my return to work had affirmed that attitude. But the tumor had done a job on me. Despite my progress, I knew that on the day the tumor was discovered, my faith in my invulnerability burned away quick, like a child's sparkler.

※

A few days after I visited the outpatient clinic, I received a letter from Dr. Tamargo. It said:

I am writing to let you know the results of the MRI scan that you underwent on September 11, 1995. This study shows no evidence of tumor residual or recurrence. I am delighted to report these results to you.

I was delighted to read them. I reached for the phone and called my parents, my daughters, some of my friends. Good news! A bona fide miracle. Maybe my brain would be good enough for the work I had to do.

The next day, on September 21, someone called about a routine mammogram that I'd had the previous week. "Saundra," she said, "we'd like for you to come in for a follow-up. The scan showed a shadow on the left breast." The earliest appointment would be at the beginning of the following week.

Calmly, I replaced the receiver. I was in my study, surrounded by the tools of the scholar—stacks of books, piles of articles to read and papers to be graded, legal pads and felt-tipped pens in my favorite colors of pink and purple. "My breast?" I asked myself, touching the left side of my chest. That little motion, soft as it was, roused an ire that had lain dormant for months, maybe since May of 1994 when I got divorced. The questions about my brain vanished. Trembling, I called Maureen. "Why is all this shit happening to me?" I yelled and cursed until I was exhausted. I don't recall what Maureen said, but over the weekend I decided that, if need be, I could live without a breast. I could not live without a brain.

The second scan revealed nothing. I was relieved, and felt confident that all was well when I visited my internist during the first week in October. My gynecologist had urged me to check on my thyroid; I was not worried because previous tests over the years had revealed nothing. Not this time. Dr. Higgs-Shipman, my new internist, found nodules when she palpated my neck; a sonogram confirmed their existence. Also, my blood pressure was elevated. She referred me to an endocrinologist, who called for a test that involved the injection of a radioactive substance. The results revealed that I had Graves' disease, characterized by an overactive thyroid gland and rapid pulse.

I decided to confine my angst over my health to Monday mornings from ten to eleven o'clock, my therapy hour with Maureen. Of course I mentioned the close calls to my friends, but I didn't go into the details of what I was feeling and why. The tumor experience had exhausted those close to me, and I was embarrassed by the soap opera my life seemed to have become. Besides, I had a faculty presentation to give in late October, meetings of the Black Women and Work seminar to attend, classes to prepare, research plans to make, and motherwork to do with Alana, then starting her junior year at UM, and Kali, who was in her last year at Hopkins. I seized the two things that I could control: what I put into my mouth and what I did with my body. I asked my endocrinologist for a diet. He said I needed to lose a few pounds to control my blood pressure and to prevent the onset of diabetes. My father had this disease, and my grandmother and aunt had died from it. The doctor gave me the diet approved by the American Diabetic Association, and I combined it with exercise, walking two miles every other day. I began losing about a pound a week.

I prepared for the faculty talk as if my job were in jeopardy—transparencies, a detailed outline with witty remarks written in the margins. The room was packed with students and colleagues. Of special importance were those who had helped me during my illness: Carol, who'd sent weekly notes on paper she'd laminated with dried flowers;

Jim, who'd kept me up to date on departmental news; Stan, who drove me to faculty meetings while I was unable to drive; Jamie, Kathy, Nathan, Brenda, and Allan, who covered my classes. As I began to talk about the characteristics of people who successfully cope in the face of stress, I relaxed. I had lived with adversity. Resilience was no longer an abstraction to me.

In October a poem came to me nearly whole, inspired by a chance encounter with an old friend. I called it "R.S.V.P." While creating it, I recalled the steady, preoperative decline in my ability to understand metaphor, or to make similes and rhymes, and the truly awful poems I wrote in the first months after surgery. I realized then that the tumor had made wordplay impossible, thereby robbing me of one of life's small pleasures. Beyond that, I'd lost the path into understanding that the act of writing gave me. With "R.S.V.P.," I seemed to have recovered craft and insight all at once. The poem told me that I'd begun to respect the larger mysteries, the life events and circumstances, good or troubling, that we can neither control nor change.

Beneath the respect, though, was the fear that I could not be effective in ways that count in the world. I was afraid that surviving was my destiny. Beyond that, I was broke. My career seemed stalled, and I no longer had the energy or the will to compete against other people or even against my own standards.

I even feared that really good things would never happen for me. I'd already reached the milestones society expected women to reach: marriage, children, a home. My life seemed to be a fragile web, spun randomly in space, with no pattern of circumstances that I could savor or anticipate with pleasure.

Rather than celebrating the small, daily wins of healing, I played and replayed an incident that happened during the eighties, when I was seeing my first therapist. In one session, I announced to her that I was engaged to be married for the second time. I spoke slowly, in flat, matter-of-fact tones about the blending of families, where the family would live, the date and time for the wedding. When I'd finished, my therapist asked gently, "But where is the joy?"

※

Until the end of the year, I tried to make it through each day without giving in to despair over my slow progress. I made a modest donation to the American Brain Tumor Association, talked with one of my students whose brother had brain cancer, resumed my visits to religious services, bought tickets to some of the "classically black" concerts of the Baltimore Symphony Orchestra, and chatted after work with Dawn, one of my daughters' friends who was living with me while she made some decisions about her life. Dawn and other members of the "posse" had waited with my daughters while I was undergoing surgery; she enjoyed telling me that she'd swooned when they glimpsed the famous pediatric neurosurgeon Ben Carson. He was operating that day. "He looked the same as he did on *60 Minutes*," Dawn reported.

At Thanksgiving, Dawn drove to Atlanta with Kali, Alana, and me. My father had a mild heart attack in early November, and we were anxious to see for ourselves that he was OK. I was skittish; around the time of his attack, news broadcasts reported that Hamilton Holmes, who along with Charlayne Hunter-Gault integrated the University of Georgia, had died of a coronary. He and Charlayne were heroes to me, as were others who wedged their way into segregated places. I was a young teenager at the start of the Civil Rights movement. My challenges were virtually invisible, such as the time I sat down at a "whites only" counter in a drugstore near my home. The waitress ignored me, and I left without a protest.

Visiting Atlanta always brought memories of a South that was still segregated when I left for college. While we were there that Thanksgiving, I thought of a poem I wanted to write; one verse would be "*We should know / your name / now, while you are here. / So many great ones depart / before we kiss them goodbye.*" I deferred the poem and visited with my mother and father and held my month-old grandniece while she slept.

I spent New Year's 1996 on my knees. Kali and I went to a midnight mass with my friend Beverly and her family. The service, in a beautiful old church in west Baltimore, was traditional with an Afrocentric flair, from the Kente cloth that the white priest wore to songs in a gospel beat. In the moments before the mass began, I mentally reviewed the year and its dismal milestones, beginning with the operation and ending with my father's heart attack as well as a biopsy for me to rule out endometrial cancer (which was thankfully negative). When we stood for the procession, I stopped trying to make mental notes, and let myself be carried along by the ritual. We joined hands during one of the prayers. Although I don't remember the words, I felt the praise, a surge of energy mingled with relief and gratitude and hope for a better year.

※

January 19, 1996, was the anniversary of my surgery, and once again I was alone. Kali had returned to her dormitory at Hopkins, Alana was spending the last few days of semester break in North Carolina, and Dawn had started a new job and moved in with friends. Throughout the day, I felt relieved and thankful that no one was ill. My fragile web, if unappealing at the moment, was at least undisturbed.

That evening, something awful happened.

The phone rang, and a hysterical caller told me that Dawn had been assaulted, stabbed more than twenty times in the head. The minute I hung up the phone, Alana called and said, "Yeah, Mom! It's been a year and nothing bad has happened." I told her about Dawn and rushed to the county hospital, but she'd been taken to a shock trauma unit in Baltimore. During her ordeal, I felt numb and helpless. Disbelieving—that kind of violence happens to other people—I stayed on the fringes: talked with her mother, comforted Kali and Alana, sent a gift. Kali's response was to go to counseling at Hopkins; between Dawn and me, she was overwhelmed. Alana coped by paying attention to her studies, her work in the dorm and at a shoe store, and her boyfriend.

During the remaining days of January and most of February, I focused on work. Within a week, the second semester started at UM, and I had a full teaching load and advisees. I met with other investigators to plan research on resilience among elementary children. The Black Women and Work seminar also resumed monthly meetings to discuss original papers; mine was scheduled for April. Also, I had the beginnings of a social life. I met a guy who eventually became a good friend, and had dinner with an old flame.

I seemed to be on automatic pilot, my feelings muted and transient as tiny waves.

Then another summons.

I got word that Eileen, one of my friends from my days at American Institutes for Research, had just had surgery for a brain tumor. The biopsy revealed that the tumor was a glioblastoma multiforme. By then, I had read enough to know that such tumors are unusually aggressive. They grow fast. Among tumors, grade IVs are the most malignant. Eileen was not doing well; friends and family were sending up prayers for her life.

During that week, I went to a Baltimore Symphony Orchestra concert and listened to each note as if I were hearing it for the first and last time in life. I couldn't imagine not being in the world to hear that music, nor could I imagine Eileen not doing the things she'd done for impoverished teens, for social workers in the new Russian republic, for political and social causes, for her daughter who was only a few years older than Alana and Kali. I thought about Dawn, whose recuperation would be emotionally, physically, and financially painful. After the concert, I cried until my eyes were swollen and my pillow damp. The tears were as much for me as they were for Eileen and Dawn. I had begun to mourn.

I think I wept, if only for a minute or two but quite often for hours, every day thereafter for the next two years. But that was my private grief. I was determined to be quietly upbeat in public and to overcome my continuing deficits. I stepped back into the roles that had served me so well before the operation. But I still tired easily; at a friend's February birthday party, I danced only once and felt so exhausted that I sat in a corner the rest of the evening. Missing a meal by even thirty minutes would leave me dizzy and stuttering. After I nearly fainted in one of my classes, I kept snacks—raisins, trail mix, juice—in my purse. I was still self-conscious about my speech. I probably made things worse by refusing to speak until I absolutely had to, or until, in the company of good friends, I felt comfortable enough. I found concentration difficult; when teaching or in meetings, the slightest noise—even the internal noise of my thought—would distract me. When I listened to a question or explanation, I had to hear with my entire mind and body. I came to see this as a good thing; you learn a lot when you pay attention.

�֍

By March 1996, I was making arrangements to conduct research under the auspices of the Center for Research on the Education of Students Placed at Risk. CRESPAR, as the center is called, was a joint project between several universities, primarily Howard, my alma mater, and Johns Hopkins. Our work there was heavily practical, "applied" research, which puts theory to work in solving educational problems. I had been doing this kind of work since my days with AIR; now I walked through the hallway of Stanton Elementary School in Washington, D.C., on my way to meet with Frances Robinson, the principal. Every time I enter a school, I temporarily revert to Saundra Rice, a little girl who looked very much like the students who sat in Stanton's classrooms. The school is in an old building like the ones that housed the schools I attended. The school mission is displayed prominently in the main hall. When I saw it, my own school's slogan, "Walk the World with Dignity," came to mind. I'm sure that was the effect our principal intended.

Ms. Robinson and I met in a room with computers sitting on tables, ready for installation. The smell of chocolate chip cookies made my stomach rumble and reminded me that lunchtime was close; parents were baking them for the PTA meeting that evening. Ms. Robinson offered me some, and the meeting began. I explained that CRESPAR wanted to examine the impact of violence on the academic life of children and to determine the circumstances under which some children were resilient and successfully adapted to school. The study would last three years. Ms. Robinson told me that her first priority was to improve students' reading and math skills; a sizable proportion of the children had scored below basic levels on a standardized test. I assured her that reading scores would be one of our main indicators of resilience. Research has shown that children who adapt successfully in the face of adversity are kids who can read and solve problems.

She would get no argument from me on the importance of reading. One of the joys of my childhood was walking to the public library—with my mother when I was very small, but alone when I was older—and selecting a big pile of books to look over before I chose the most tempting ones to check out. I was intrigued with just about everything but fish, which I feared and avoided assiduously. When I was a teenager and had been told that my fears were irrational, I went to the library and tried to find a book on the phobia. Just as many kids today turn to the computer for answers, I turned to books and still do. I nodded my head in agreement when Ms. Robinson said, "We're doing a disservice to our students if we can't teach them to read!"

She further explained that many of the students had been exposed to drugs before they were born and had great problems in the classroom. And practically all of the students were poor and from single-parent homes. "What can you do to help the teachers deal with the conditions of the children's lives?" she asked. Later, when I talked to teachers, the same question arose. One teacher put it bluntly: "We don't need another researcher coming in, getting publications at our expense, and moving on. We need help for these students." It was clear to me that I would not be doing an "objective" study, one in which I could maintain my distance. I offered what I could on my budget: information to teachers for their own development as professionals; support for the school's outreach to parents; and assistance gathering and analyzing data on students' self-concepts, reasons for wanting to read, and other potential strengths.

While I waited for word on whether Stanton would collaborate with CRESPAR, I kept in contact with friends who gave me updates on Eileen's condition. It was a strange feeling, being among the healthy, yet anxious about the life of a person who was in the same situation that I had been in just twelve months ago. Eileen pulled through the postoperative crisis, and went home. In late March I accompanied her to one of her radiation treatments. We talked about Decadron and Tegretol and pushed aside our hair to reveal the scars. She marveled that I didn't have to undergo chemotherapy and radiation; she would begin chemo shortly. During one conversation about the incredible coincidence of our illness, she asked, "Saundra, we both worked hard, raised wonderful children, tried to be kind, and what did we get?" "Brain tumors," I said, and we held hands, laughing and crying.

�֎

After speaking with parents and conferring with Ms. Robinson a few more times, I finished the semester with a favorable decision from Stanton. I presented a draft of my personal history of resilience at the Black Women and Work meeting to very encouraging reviews. But I was still ambivalent about my classes. I enjoyed working with students one-on-one and in small groups, but I had difficulty presenting lively lectures. I still relied heavily on my notes; there was little spontaneity. The students' evaluations gave me mixed reviews. I rated high on knowledge of my discipline, but how I taught what I knew was another story.

That May, the old AIR gang had lunch with Eileen at a restaurant in the renovated Union Station in Washington, and Kali graduated from Hopkins with honors, a Phi Beta Kappa key, and enough credits to earn her B.A. and master's in history. She also wore silver shoes and big, dangling, heart-shaped silver earrings. Those shiny touches reminded me of both daughters' steely determination to meet their educational goals and look out for me at the same time. Kali decided to follow in the footsteps of her paternal grandfather, the late Donald Gaines Murray Sr. He attended the University of Maryland law school after a successful suit in 1938, *Murray v. Maryland*, which Thurgood Marshall argued before the U.S. Supreme Court. He was shunned throughout his years at Maryland, ignored by professors and students alike.

Nearly three decades later, his granddaughter was off to Duke University on a scholarship. As she entered the big canopy on the Hopkins quadrangle, Alana and I waved and called her name. She grinned, and marched to the podium, where she sat with the Hopkins president and President George Bush. I was sure that Kali would be just fine. I'd brought plenty of tissues, but I was dry-eyed. I didn't want to miss a thing.

※

By early fall 1996, I had taken my first airplane trips since the operation. I'd dreaded flying again; given my luck, I expected there'd be an accident. Or maybe the air pressure would make my brain explode through my scar. One of these imagined catastrophes was highly unlikely, and the other was downright irrational, but my fears distorted my thoughts as reliably as my reading glasses magnified words. After the plane reached maximum altitude, I took a deep breath. My brain stayed in place. I began to enjoy the ride to California. One trip was to the American Sports Institute in Marin County, where my doctoral student and I were setting up a study of a school program called Promoting Achievement in School Through Sport, or PASS. We met with the developers of PASS, and they described how the program fostered resilience by helping kids transfer the skills learned in sports to the challenges of academic mastery. My mood brightened when I tried out some of the physical exercises; I walked a mile or two each day, and I had the best chocolate dessert one evening at dinner. I was optimistic and feeling healthy by the time I made the second part of my journey to Harvard for a presentation at the

Principal's Center. I'd worked on my talk for weeks; I recall only minor glitches and told myself that things had gone very well indeed.

In September 1996, Alana started her senior year at UM. Kali was in Durham. My classes resumed, and I seemed to be better at remembering facts and names. I assisted Stanton with staff development and did the chores that went with setting up a research study. The Black Women and Work group had its first meeting: we would be planning a spring conference. I had my annual MRI and conference with Dr. Tamargo. He was clearly pleased at the results of the scan, which showed that my brain was still healing. Things seemed to be settling down, although no amount of prayer, meditation, or affirmation could still the voice that warned, "Anything can happen."

※

A friend called in October to tell me that Eileen's condition had suddenly worsened. By the end of the month, she lay dying in a hospice. I saw her once more the night before she passed. She was not conscious, but I followed her daughter's lead and stroked her hand and spoke softly about shared memories. Her memorial service was on a sunny November day, and her partner read from the diary Eileen had kept during her illness. Although I wondered, "Why did she die? Why did I live?" when I heard her words, she was alive again if only for a moment. I don't recall them exactly, but the sense of the message was in a letter that Eileen had written and misplaced. It was found after she died, and her daughter sent it at Christmas to all of Eileen's friends. The letter told the story of her illness: the sudden loss of vision and memory, waking up to a grim prognosis after brain surgery, the abundant support of family and friends. "So what's to come?" she wrote. "Who knows. We live with the uncertainty and plan and hope for the best."

Those words would become my mantra, my formula to dispel the survivor's guilt, regret, and self-doubt that visited the space left by the tumor. I was aware that negative thinking impeded healing, and was determined to follow Eileen's example of optimism. Perhaps because of this, I felt good about Christmas that year. All of us—my daughters, parents, brother and sister-in-law, nephew and nieces—gathered at my sister's home in Atlanta for dinner. Alana filmed a documentary of the occasion. She asked each person the same question: what are you grateful for? Life, health, each other, being together were the answers.

✲

Six days into 1997, I turned fifty. My daughters and I went to Barbara's house, and we had dinner and cake with her, her husband, Jim, and their two children. I've never been one to insist that people mark the occasion of my birth, perhaps because my birthday comes just twelve days after Christmas. At times I've been downright rude when people did things for me. On my thirtieth birthday, I arrived at work to find a big banner announcing that fact. I tore down the sign, thanking the person who was thoughtful enough to remember me but letting her know that I preferred private celebrations. But as I blew out the five candles on the cake that Barbara baked, one for each decade, I told myself, "I may not have everything I want in life, but I am alive."

Later in the week, I decided I'd had enough of the off-white walls in my house, went to a hardware store and bought seven gallons of paint, got on a ladder for the first time in years, and went to work. My friends know how I love to decorate, but I'd done little more in my house than arrange the furniture when we'd moved there six months before the diagnosis. The painting took a couple of weeks, but by the time it was done, Alana's bedroom had become buttercream; mine, soft mauve; and my study, rosy beige. I bought a quilt for Kali's room, which we'd painted blue before I got sick, hung the pictures that had been stacked in corners for almost three years, and rearranged my collection of miniature houses. I have always been intrigued by Jung's notion that the house is the symbol of the self, and now I see that in giving my house a new look, I started giving myself a new way to look at life.

When I returned to campus after the semester break, I taught my spring courses and became better at mixing different kinds of activities within the three-hour blocks that the classes met. Sometimes, students lingered to chat with me after classes or dropped by my office unexpectedly to talk; I liked that and took it as a sign that things were improving. Data collection at Stanton went smoothly, and Ms. Robinson and I began a dialogue on how emphasizing kids' strengths, instead of their deficiencies, could transform the way the school regarded instruction and the students themselves. In April, I attended an educational conference and on the way stopped in Detroit and visited with Fran and her husband.

At the end of the semester, Kali and I watched Alana graduate with honors in government and politics from UM. Although Alana had first attempted to enter UM's business school and then switched majors, she eventually decided to pursue the plans she announced in a newspaper profile that appeared when she was a senior in high school: "She plans to become a teacher and educational philosopher." With a scholarship in hand, she was on her way to Brown University to work on her master of arts in teaching. Her grandmothers were especially delighted; both are retired public school teachers.

People began asking me, how did you do it—rear two delightful young women who are smart, assertive, and down-to-earth? My response: I and all the rest of the family loved them, allowed them to make decisions appropriate to their abilities and let them experience the consequences, encouraged their spiritual progress, took it for granted that they would do their best (whether or not their best was the highest or fastest or most of anything) in school, listened to their accounts of what they did each day, read to them (their father went through all the *Chronicles of Narnia* before they were five, and books by Eloise Greenfield were favorites), took them to the library as often as they wanted to go, and made room for their friends in our homes. Sometimes we had fun. All the rest—the ballet lessons, the vacations to interesting places, the summer enrichment activities—were good things. But what I think was essential conforms to the conditions that researcher Bonnie Benard, writing on the topic of resilience, found to be vital in environments that protect kids against the stresses of life: caring and support, high expectations, and opportunities to participate.

꙰

That summer I worked on my research, dated an eternal bachelor, and took golf lessons. I am no athlete, so I was thrilled when I actually starting hitting golf balls consistently and in the correct form. When my daughters and I went to Atlanta in August to see the family, all of us gathered on my parents' lawn and had a grand old time swinging the golf clubs I'd brought down in the trunk of my car. Despite some irksome problems that doctors had attributed to the surgery—a damaged optic nerve and tinnitus (ringing in the ears)— my body felt strong for the first time in years.

It turned out that my brain was healing properly, too, as confirmed by my annual MRI and consultation with Dr. Tamargo in September. By then, two and a half years had passed since my surgery. I was still trying to piece together what happened to me, and I'd brought a list of questions: How does the brain recover? What surgical procedures were used in my operation? What causes the tears after brain surgery? What questions did the residents ask me on rounds? What did these questions reveal?

Dr. Tamargo answered each one in detail, in plain language. In response to the one about the questions residents asked me, Dr. Tamargo surprised me by commenting, "We weren't sure we could save your ability to speak and write." Until then, I had no idea that the outcome of my surgery was in any way doubtful. Had he mentioned it when I was fresh out of surgery, I might have become discouraged.

I checked my watch. Forty or so minutes had passed since my appointment began, and I thought, "You need to hurry up and get out of here. He's a busy man and has other people to see." But when I glanced at him, he was in a quiet, expectant pose, perhaps waiting for me to finish the list of questions. I realized that at every stage in my recovery, friends and professionals alike had admonished me to slow down. They said things will get better, time heals all wounds. By his patient attention, Dr. Tamargo provided a model for me.

✺

Life for me that fall of 1997 settled into a routine mixed-bag of a life. I taught one class that semester and spent the released time on my research at Stanton. Alana was in her second semester at Brown; Kali was a second-year law student at Duke. For the first time since they were born, I had the house to myself for long periods of time.

My spells of weeping continued. I suspected that the cause had changed from mourning about the specific events—Eileen's death, Dawn's assault, my empty nest, and the lingering memories of illness—to a more pervasive sense of loss. There were reminders everywhere of what used to be. Over lunch with a married friend, I might regret that I was alone except for the occasional date. When colleagues talked about their latest books and articles, I mentally reviewed the months since I'd written anything and wondered whether I'd be further along in my once-promising career if the tumor had been diagnosed sooner. I hungered for accounts that explained the crazy behavior and symptoms I displayed when the tumor was growing—anything that would help me to recreate the chain of events that led to my current circumstances. More often than not, I found research on animals or on other conditions, like alcoholism and Alzheimer's. Occasionally I would stumble on an article that was relevant. One of them mentioned a study that compared normal people with patients who suffered damage to their frontal lobes from tumors or strokes. The researchers discovered that the patients fared very nicely on verbal and memory tasks, but these same patients made huge blunders in real-life decisions involving finances and social relations. "Like the ones I'd made," I thought, remembering the missteps guided by the same tumorous mind that produced, until the last months before my operation, articles in social scientific journals.

I realize now that information was not all I sought. I wanted something that would compensate for my losses. When I first came home from the hospital, I just wanted an acknowledgement of error from the doctors who had failed to detect the tumor or follow up on my symptoms. My friends had other ideas. "This is a slam-dunk case," one declared. "You went to the emergency room barely able to talk. Someone should have given you a CAT scan or an MRI or even an EKG, not Valium." Everyone seemed to agree that the internist I consulted after the May 1994 trip to the emergency room should have checked, as he said he would, the records from that visit. "With your symptoms, he needed to refer you to a neurologist."

The lawyer I consulted in May 1995 had, like my friends, urged me to file a lawsuit. I retained him, but nearly three years passed and basic actions, such as getting medical records, had not been completed. Hounding the attorney was not my main priority; healing was. By October 1997, Kali reminded me that the statute of limitations would soon run out, and I needed to decide whether to go forward or quit. Kali, then in her second year at law school, was skeptical about whether I had a good claim, but she was against legal action from the start. "Mom, I don't want to see you go through the scrutiny. The lawyers for the hospital will grill you on your psychiatric history and do their best to discredit you. You've already been through enough."

That was true, but a cash settlement would go a long way toward making my life a little less stressful. More than that, I knew that I needed actively to explore all the possibilities. If I hadn't been able to be my own best advocate while I was ill, I could certainly do that now. Thinking that I needed other opinions, I consulted two top malpractice attorneys. Both said I had to meet three criteria: there had to be damages (I had those); someone had to have goofed up (someone did); and my treatment had to be more serious than if the tumor had been diagnosed earlier (it was not). Surgical removal of the kind of tumor I had is the standard treatment. In November, a month before the statute of limitations ran out, I put aside any thoughts I might have had for a legal remedy. Despite my ambivalence about a malpractice suit, I was disappointed and sad.

Some losses are irreparable.

※

My customary response to the realization that something I once had and valued greatly was gone forever was a long period of depression, fatigue, the slide down the sides of the hole I seemed to dwell in those years before the tumor was removed. I braced myself for the arrival of another dark night of the soul. To my relief and surprise, it did not come. For three years I'd seen life as a struggle that I had to transcend. But over the summer, I'd begun to have moments of pleasure and fun; my family and friends were doing well, I was enjoying my work, and I looked forward to Thanksgiving with my daughters. On November 4, I wrote in my diary:

Today I decided to give myself the gift of one year without struggle. I will explore—try things out.

❈

If they are lucky, children of divorce get to spend holidays with both parents. Over the years since their father and I had separated, Kali and Alana had settled into a routine. The main Thanksgiving meal was spent with one of us, dessert with the other. Christmas Eve and morning with their father; Christmas afternoon with me.

For Thanksgiving 1997, I prepared a big, traditional feast, including the oyster dressing beloved by Baltimoreans. Alana flew in from Providence, and Kali drove up from Durham with two of her friends. The conversation at dinner was lively and passionate. I listened as these four very bright and articulate young adults shared with me their hopes for having an impact on the world through law, education, biotechnology, and biochemistry. I surprised myself by declaring, "For almost three decades much of my work has been devoted to closing the gap in attainment created by race, gender, and class." I'd not said that aloud for years. I talked about my writing on psychology of black women, about my work at AIR, UPO, and Hopkins, my consulting practice in evaluating programs aimed at increasing minority access to careers in science, math, and technology, and how my underlying mission linked all these disparate areas. I thought, "And I still want and like to do this."

From then on, work as I defined it became a refuge from the inevitable disappointments, setbacks, and struggles that happen to everyone who lives long enough. I shifted my focus from the products of work—in my case, the publications, course evaluations, and grant applications—to working itself. I figured that the works would come in the process of doing things that were useful to others and at the same time enjoyable for me. At Stanton, Ms. Robinson and I started mapping the school's resources along two dimensions in a resilience strategy: reducing the risks to children in the environment, and building a safety net of academic, family, and community services to protect them. I began to look at the research data with an eye toward the most effective way to tell a story of the school's efforts to improve students' success in reading and math. I continued my search for effective ways to present ideas and evidence to my students in classes, using information from the Center for Excellence in Teaching in UM's College of Education and tips from Alana, who advised me to learn every student's name and what they wanted most from their educational experience. Examining my own life story in the essay I was writing for the Black Women and Work project prompted me to explore the ways that identity is formed through stories about ourselves. I began to outline future research that would examine resilience in black women's autobiographical writings.

Amid these joyful moments, each day I still wept. I had reduced my bitching and moaning about loss to my therapy hour and to occasional, seemingly normal outbursts in front of my closest friends and daughters. The tumor and its aftermath were no longer foremost in my conscious awareness. I could not understand the source of my continuing tears.

But analytical methods are not the only paths to truth. Seymour Epstein, whose theory and research is on personality psychology, describes dual ways of knowing, the rational and the experiential.

About the rational mode he says, "It is a very inefficient system for responding to everyday events, and its long term adaptability remains to be tested. (It may yet lead to the destruction of all life on our planet)." On the experiential, he comments that "it is a source of intuitive wisdom and creativity."[1] This mind system represents events as vivid images, but the experiential mind can also use narratives, scripts, and metaphor, the basic tool of the poet.

As usual, the dreamer in me knew what the rational me could not. During the first quarter of 1998, three nightmares punctuated the otherwise happy activities of my nocturnal brain. The first one came in January. I made a one-line note about it in my diary, but the details are fixed in my mind because in the dream I am drowning, a fate that scares me more than the thought of fish. I am in the water because someone grabbed my purse and I ran from the thief and jumped in.

The second nightmare came on March 13, and I wrote the scene in my diary:

I was at a party in a vast house that one of my friends owned. I wandered from room to room, meeting another friend and looking for my date, who'd disappeared. I went outside (the front yard was a rural scene—complete with dogs and chickens) & my car was gone even though I still had my keys in my pocket.

I recorded the last dream on April 13:

Dreamed that I left my house unlocked to go for a walk. Something told me to go back and I found someone there. She was stealing &

drank tea calmly from my teapot. I flung hot water on her and when
she retaliated in kind I dared her to run. She went into the kitchen
and killed someone. I tried to call 911 & she struggled with me.

I awoke sobbing, but when my tears subsided, I felt a space open wide in my mind. After that, I stopped talking about the tumor so much, blaming it for every negative experience since adolescence and all my struggles since the operation. Although Dr. Tamargo told me that during the surgery only a small section had been preserved for biopsy, I imagined the tumor whole somewhere, imprisoned, life-less, in a jar where it could no longer reach me. My daily habit of weeping diminished gradually.

Later that summer, I made sense of those dreams prompted by a conversation I had with one of the women in the Black Women and Work seminar. I was meeting with a small group of the members in July 1998; we were critiquing chapters each of us had submitted for the book that was the culminating project of the seminar. Besides me, three others sat in the comfortable sofas in the basement of the house where we gathered. The conversation was open and easy; we pointed out what we liked in each paper, and then focused on passages we didn't understand or on things that could be added or omitted. We laughed sometimes; ideas flowed. As in the larger seminar, this work-ing group mixed criticism with friendly support, a style the project had fostered over the three years.

We turned to my paper, an abridged version of one of the chap-ters of my story, and after I got feedback on strengths and weaknesses, we talked about what it means to have a diseased brain. The conversation was not abstract, not intellectual. One of our mothers had Alzheimer's; one of us had had a stroke. Eventually, we moved on to lighter topics, but not before one of my sister scholars turned to me and said, "Saundra, when you first joined the seminar I thought, Oh, she just doesn't have much to say. Now I think I saw you healing, right before our eyes."

A few days later I was at a writers' retreat, and the meaning of the dreams came to me. The thief was the tumor. It nearly killed me in the first dream. In the second, the tumor/thief got one thing, my car, which I owned, but I was alive and still had the key. In the final dream, I fought back and called for help.

Those dreams echo the story of my illness and healing. Years passed as the tumor grew from a tiny mass to the orange-sized glob that Dr. Tamargo and Dr. Oshiro removed. Along the way, the tumor took my ability to describe the world, to communicate with people in it, and to understand my experience of it. I surmise that my narrative, my story, disintegrated: from whole connected paragraphs linked by plot and theme to sentences and phrases, and finally to wordless emotions.

As the second dream revealed, I survived. The tumor got away with some of what I had, but enough of me remained to write a few words and phrases and begin a new poem. The story of my struggle to stabilize my physical and intellectual foundation was told in the days when I rested while others cared for me, when I walked beside the little lake in my neighborhood, when I learned to pay attention to all sorts of stimuli in speech therapy, and when I tried to recover enough brain power to do my work as a scholar. As a black woman, I was all too familiar with the survival narrative; for many of us, it is the only story we know—how to get from day to day.

But in reentering the world beyond my wisteria trellis, I went beyond loss and survival to a new narrative. It is built on the two fundamental human tendencies that psychologists and others have identified. One is agency, expressed in strivings for power and independence. In my dream, I fought back. In my life, I was trying to master the art of teaching, to recapture my work as a thinker through the sisterly exchange of ideas and critique in the Black Women and Work project, and to recreate my identity as a scholar through my research in schools.

The other motivational theme is connection, the strivings for love and intimacy. In my dream, I called for help. It came from my family and friends, from Ms. Robinson and the teachers at Stanton, from Dr. Tamargo and Maureen, from my sister scholars in the Black Women and Work project.

※

Life stories of adults who have overcome adversity or unforeseen calamities are the basis for descriptions of resilience as transformation. These stories describe stress and trauma that precipitate fundamental shifts. These changes can be in the quality of relationships from abusive to empathic. The ways you see yourself and the world can also shift. In the months before the tumor was diagnosed, I had little awareness of actively coping. My identity, my sense of a person inside my head who asked, "What's going on?" and "What do I do about it?" then acted accordingly, was unreliable, becoming progressively disabled. I could not think of options, plan, or carry out strategies. Illness and other life changes not only disrupted my coping but depleted the resources I needed to manage stress. When

I changed jobs, I went from a place in which I'd worked for six years and developed strong bonds with colleagues to another environment in which I knew only one person. I was newly divorced as well; my connections with my former husband's family had been severed. Illness further alienated me. I was too fatigued to do normal things, such as shop for groceries or make routine phone calls to family members and friends.

Before the tumor was removed, and perhaps because it was on my brain, the sheer force of habit and the expectations of other people carried me along from day to day. Put me in a situation, with all the relevant cues, and I did the right things, if only minimally, in my social roles as mother, daughter, colleague, friend. I could not count on my feelings. At times I would react with anger to kind words, or say the first thing that popped into my mind, whether it fit the occasion or not. The physical world, particularly my body, was unstable as well.

My transformation began during the time I spent alone after my mother returned to Atlanta. I began reading stories written by persons who had encounters with catastrophic illness, and at the same time started to piece together the events and circumstances of the illness that led to the traumatic moment of finding out that I had a brain tumor.

Telling my story gave me a way of accepting loss and regaining perspective and a sense of connection to others and everything around me. I had many safe places, not only in which to recount events as I experienced them but also in which to express the feelings I had. I wrote poems and this book. I told my friends who hadn't been able to see for themselves; I spoke to a class that was studying brain functions; the topic recurred in therapy hours; and people who had relatives with brain tumors wanted to know about symptoms. With my friend Eileen, the telling was mutual. More important as Alana pointed out, people actually listened to me, something that she doubted happened as much as it could. I find it remarkable that during my illness I didn't lose the awareness I could voice my concerns and feelings and that somebody would listen to me and not punish me for what I said.

Looking back to my childhood, I find that I've always had these "zones of narrative safety," as my daughters and I call these sites of expression and listening. I had family members, the recreation center where I danced and sang to recordings of fairy tales, the librarian who required me to report on all the books I claimed to read for a valuable certificate. All of them helped me to create my narrative.

If identity, as many scholars now construe it, is the story you tell about yourself, then a safety zone where you can exercise the power of expression any way you choose may be one of the elements necessary for weaving trauma and adversity into the vast web of life, putting them in a place where you can see them for what they took and what they gave. Each time I told my story or read or heard another's, I gained new insights that guided my thoughts and actions. The many small epiphanies seemed to add up to these lessons: While you may have support, ultimately you are in charge of your recovery. Even if death or permanent disability is likely, try as hard as you can to restore your physical self, your social and mental competence, and your sense of dignity. Do this by any compassionate means available. Be graceful and courteous in vulnerability; people who care for you have feelings and needs of their own, and your adversity distresses them, too. Do things now because they're right and healthy and kind, not because there will be a possible payoff in the future.

※

It is November 1998. Alana and I are in my car. We listen to *Ike and Tina Turner's Greatest Hits*. The song "Proud Mary" comes up first. It brings back a memory from the summer in Atlanta when my family played golf on the front lawn. We had put away the clubs and gone into my parents' house. I suppose the spirit of fun and the joy of being together as a family just carried us along, and we put on some music. With my sister behind the camcorder and the family clapping in time, the girls and I did our rendition of "Proud Mary." Whirling and lip-synching, the girls were the Ikettes, I was Tina, and my grand-niece, then about two, was a free spirit doing her own dance.

I think that marked the moment when I understood that resilience is more than surviving, more than regaining physical and mental competence. It is also the process of recovering spirit and will, faith, anger, sadness, and above all, joy. I'd experienced the miracle of Psalm 30:11: "Thou hast turned for me my mourning into dancing; thou hast put off my sackcloth, and girded me with gladness."

Epilogue: Courtesy of My Right Brain

I walk through the revolving doors of the Johns Hopkins outpatient clinic, stop at the counter to my left, and show the receptionist my orange ID card. She checks my name on the appointment sheet and tells me to go the third floor. I check in at "Advanced Imaging/MRI" and sit in one of the black vinyl seats that define the waiting areas lining the corridor.

It is August 24, 1999, and this will be my first scan in two years. When the technician fetches me, I feel no need to follow him. I know the drill. Go to the locker. Remove all metal and place your extraneous stuff in the cubicle. Use the bathroom. Return to the room that houses the MRI. Position yourself on the movable table.

The technician tells me they've reduced the time needed for the scans. I will have one that lasts two minutes, followed by a second one of four minutes. I will come out of the machine to receive an injection of dye, and then the third scan will be six minutes, followed by the last one of three minutes.

Everything's cool until I realize that I've forgotten to take an antianxiety medication. I will have to endure the scan with the music that is piped into the machine and the passages from the Bible that I've recited during previous scans. I manage to make it through the first set of scans, but I am trembling violently when I am rolled out for the injection.

"This reminds me of the worst time of my life," I say, tears welling in my eyes. "Memories can be powerful," the technician says, "but you're not back there now. You're here." I take a deep breath, and say, "Thank you."

The rest of the scan is fine, and I pass the time before my appointment with Dr. Tamargo looking at the exhibit on display. Today, there's one with early X-ray equipment: glass plates, tubing, and the like. The accompanying scientific article is dated October 1951. I think, "Would an X-ray have shown my tumor? Would Dr. Tamargo have known the precise location?" I think of all the centuries that passed before doctors were able to treat the brain under safe conditions, and I am grateful for MRIs.

Next, I go to the fifth floor, to "Neurology/Neurosurgery." Dr. Tamargo greets me, and asks if I have any problems with muscle weakness. I say no, and then respond to his question about medications I am taking. "Your speech has recovered completely," he says, smiling. He goes to retrieve my scans from Imaging, and returns, again smiling.

"Looks great. Terrific. No sign of recurrence."

We chat about our work for a few moments. I tell him about Eileen, and he mentions work he has done to prolong life with the type of tumor that she had. As for me, he says the chances of my tumor returning are very, very small.

�֎

I would love to know what went on in my head as I regained what I needed for the life I enjoy today. Although I must adhere to one or two more rounds of postoperative monitoring, I don't dwell on the small possibility of a recurrence. I choose to direct my thoughts to positive things: Alana loves her job as a high school teacher; Kali is now working in a law firm; Dawn has completed her training as a licensed practical nurse. At this moment my mother and friends are doing well, but my father, who is diabetic, is "ailing," he says.

I am still rebuilding my life. I fight occasional blues whose source is self-doubt or regret; I wonder at times if the years while the tumor grew left indelible traces, hard mental habits to break. I am more comfortable writing than speaking aloud, but I have come a long way from the person who could talk but couldn't organize her mind well enough to recite the letters of the alphabet. Now, I am planning studies to see if some of my hunches about how resilience works apply to others; I am particularly intrigued with how people experience community throughout their lives. I have recommitted myself to efforts to improve education for students who face multiple impediments to success. I laugh more easily and enjoy my time with good friends. My spiritual practice brings me feelings of strength and peace.

I don't remember things as well as I'd like, so I jot down phone numbers, sentences that I want to incorporate in my papers, lists of the three things I need from the grocery store, titles of CDs I'd like to buy. I sketch arrangements for my collection of miniature houses, and I gather fabric swatches and paint chips to improve my memory of colors. Just as I did while in speech therapy, I am honing the skills I need to concentrate, store information, and recall things when I need them. Sometimes the textures, smells, sounds, and sights I sense trigger similar fragments stored in my brain.

On one of those occasions, I recalled some of the details of that August day in 1994, when I wandered, tumor and all, among my relatives at the Weems Family Reunion. I feel the heat, which is so intense that it instantly dries the moisture that rings my hairline. I stumble once or twice on patches of red dirt, cracked and dry, which show through grass still green despite the hint of drought. I feel the pressure of my father's hands, gnarled with arthritis, as he leads me from one relative to the next. "Do you remember Saundra, my first-born?" he asks. "When she was just a tiny thing, she used to sit out on the porch, swinging and talking to great-grandmama, a sweet old lady talking with a sweet little girl."

I have no idea what I, as a toddler of three, talked about with Carrie Weems, my great-great-grandmother who was over ninety when I knew her. The images that remain of her are her farm and the plants that grew there. The cotton resisted tiny fingers that tried to pull it from the bolls, and the muscadine grapes tasted too sharp for an unsophisticated palate. Those faint images are part of my story now. I remember them.

Notes

Prologue

1. I discuss three meanings of resilience. For explanations of the brain's resilience, see Donald G. Stein, Simon Brailowsky, and Bruno Will, *Brain Repair* (New York: Oxford University Press, 1995). The authors offer five explanations of recovery: (1) the brain has a back-up system that takes over damaged functions; (2) brain cells have equipotentiality, the ability of individual healthy cells to do the work of damaged cells; (3) functional substitution occurs when parts of the brain not associated with a specific job retool to do the work of damaged parts; (4) with time, deficits following injury can return to normal, provided that the injury is not of a severe type; and (5) unused parts of the brain do the work of damaged parts.

The views I discuss pertaining to psychological resilience come from several sources. For a discussion of the three phenomena commonly referred to as psychological resilience, see Ann S. Masten, Karen M. Best, and Norman Garmezy, "Resilience and Development: Contributions from the Study of Children Who Overcome Adversity," *Development and Psychopathology* 2, no. 4 (1990): 425–44. Studies also suggest that protective processes contribute to resilience. These are processes that promote competence in adverse as well as favorable circumstances and include intellectual functioning, relationships with caring adults, and the self-regulation of attention, feelings, and actions. In resilient children, one or more of these processes have continued to function despite an unfavorable environment. See Ann S. Masten and J. Douglas Coatsworth, "The Development of Competence in Favorable and Unfavorable Environments: Lessons from Research on Successful Children," *American Psychologist* 53, no. 2 (1998): 205–20; and Michael Rutter, "Psychosocial Resilience and Protective Mechanisms," *American Journal of Orthopsychiatry* 57, no. 3 (1987): 316–31.

My understanding of resilience as transformation was enriched by reading Pamela LePage-Lees, *From Disadvantaged Girls to Successful Women: Education and Women's Resiliency* (Westport: Praeger, 1997), and Carol E. Franz and Abigail J. Stewart, eds., *Women Creating Lives: Identities, Resilience, and Resistance* (Boulder: Westview, 1994).

You Are Different Now

1. "Like other brain tumors, the cause of meningiomas is unknown. Researchers are studying several theories. However, an abnormal chromosome (#22) is the most common abnormality in meningiomas. But, what causes this chromosomal abnormality is uncertain." American Brain Tumor Association, *About Meningioma* (Chicago, 1992): 2.

2. For a history of medicine in cultural context, see Roy Porter, *The Greatest Benefit to Mankind: A Medical History of Humanity* (New York: W. W. Norton, 1998). For a journalistic account of neurological medicine, see David Noonan, *Neuro-: Life on the Frontlines of Brain Surgery and Neurological Medicine* (New York: Simon and Schuster, 1989).

Nourished on Nightmare

1. National Institute of Neurological Disorders and Stroke, "Brain and Spinal Cord Tumors: Hope Through Research" (Washington, D.C.: U.S. Government Printing Office, 1993): 10.

Witnesses

1. Stein, Brailowsky, and Will, *Brain Repair,* 78.

Recovering Work

1. Social support is a resource that has been studied extensively in adults and children. Social support is defined in many ways, but measures of the concept can focus on the presence or absence of interpersonal relationships; the frequency with which we make contact with others; our perceptions of support from family, friends, or others outside the family; or the actual types of resources we get (such as money, love and caring, information, and time).

2. Oliver Sacks, "A Matter of Identity," in *The Man Who Mistook His Wife for a Hat and Other Clinical Tales* (New York: Harper Perennial, 1985): 110.

Mourning into Dancing

1. Seymour Epstein, "Integration of the Cognitive and the Psychodynamic Unconscious," *American Psychologist* 49, no. 8 (1994): 715.

Bibliography

American Brain Tumor Association. *A Primer of Brain Tumors: A Patient's Reference Manual*. Des Plains, Ill., n.d.

———. *About Meningioma*. Chicago, 1992.

Benard, Bonnie. *Fostering Resiliency in Kids: Protective Factors in the Family, School, and Community*. Portland: Western Center for Drug-Free Schools and Communities, 1991.

Brooks, Gwendolyn. "Annie Allen." In *Selected Poems*. New York: Harper & Row, 1963.

Epstein, Seymour. "Integration of the Cognitive and the Psychodynamic Unconscious." *American Psychologist* 49, no. 8 (1994): 709–24.

Franz, Carol E., and Abigail J. Stewart, eds. *Women Creating Lives: Identities, Resilience, and Resistance*. Boulder: Westview, 1994.

Golden, Daniel. "Building a Better Brain." *Life*, July 1994, 62–70.

House, Ernest R. *Jesse Jackson and the Politics of Charisma: The Rise and Fall of the PUSH/EXCEL Program*. Boulder: Westview, 1988.

LePage-Lees, Pamela. *From Disadvantaged Girls to Successful Women: Education and Women's Resiliency*. Westport: Praeger, 1997.

Masten, Ann S., Karin M. Best, and Norman Garmezy. "Resilience and Development: Contributions from the Study of Children Who Overcome Adversity." *Development and Psychopathology* 2, no. 4 (1991): 425–44.

Masten, Ann S., and J. Douglas Coatsworth. "The Development of Competence in Favorable and Unfavorable Environments: Lessons from Research on Successful Children." *American Psychologist* 53, no. 2 (1998): 205–20.

National Institute of Neurological Disorders and Stroke. *Brain and Spinal Cord Tumors: Hope Through Research*. Washington, D.C.: U.S. Government Printing Office, 1993.

Noonan, David. *Neuro-: Life on the Frontlines of Brain Surgery and Neurological Medicine*. New York: Simon and Schuster, 1989.

Oliver, Mary. "Dogfish." In *Dream Work*. New York: Atlantic Monthly, 1986.

Porter, Roy. *The Greatest Benefit to Mankind: A Medical History of Humanity*. New York: W. W. Norton, 1998.

Rutter, Michael. "Psychosocial Resilience and Protective Mechanisms," *American Journal of Orthopsychiatry* 57, no. 3 (1987): 316–31.

Sacks, Oliver. "A Matter of Identity." In *The Man Who Mistook His Wife for a Hat and Other Clinical Tales*. New York: Harper Perennial, 1985.

Stein, Donald G., Simon Brailowsky, and Bruno Will. *Brain Repair*. New York: Oxford University Press, 1995.

Walcott, Derek. *The Odyssey: A Stage Version*. New York: Farrar Straus Giroux, 1993.

Washington, Mary Helen. "On Discovering Self and Empowerment in Black Women's Literature." In *My Soul Is a Witness: African-American Women's Spirituality*. Edited by Gloria Wade-Gayles. Boston: Beacon, 1995.

Acknowledgments

I hope that the deep affection and gratitude I feel for my family, friends, and colleagues came through in these pages. I called many of these individuals by name; others will recognize themselves in the many kind deeds they performed.

I lived to tell this story because two extraordinarily gifted healers—Dr. Rafael Tamargo, neurosurgeon, and Maureen Kehoe, psychotherapist—cared about me as a whole person. I appreciate them, as well as Dr. Eric Oshiro, the nurses on Meyer Nine, and the therapists at Horizon Health and Rehabilitation.

Special thanks to all who went beyond the call of friendship: Barbara Wasik and James Byrnes, Frances and Warren Young, Marcia and Bob Gorrie, Beverly and Howard Henderson, Jamie Metsala, Rosa Walker Murray, Kathy Murray, Patricia Rice Murphy, Gary and Denise Gottfredson, Carol Seefeldt, Barbara McHugh, Albertha and James Workman, Karen Porter, Sue Fradkin, Janet Felsten, Seth and Pearlena Patters, Francis Robinson, Stan Bennett, Dee Thompson, and my neighbors in Columbia, Md. I am indebted beyond words to each of you.

I relied on the encouragement and friendly criticism from fellow writers in Jeffrey's House Party, the Deepdene Writers' Workshop, and The Life Writing Project at the University of Maryland. My sister scholars in the Black Women and Work seminar and my students nurtured my return to an intellectual community and championed this project. The seminar and the University of Maryland Consortium on Research on Race, Gender, and Ethnicity, both funded by the Ford Foundation, provided support for the writing and preparation of portions of this manuscript. Lisa Crye, Margaret Osburn, Mary Helen Washington, the late John Hollifield, Alana Murray, and Kali Murray gave me valuable editorial suggestions on various drafts. With good humor, Elizabeth Willis provided fine technical support.

My colleagues at the University of Maryland were incredibly patient, understanding that there were duties I could not easily undertake and quietly arranging to spread the load. The former and current chairs of my department—professors Robert Hardy and Stephen Porges, respectively—showed compassion throughout my recovery. Many people kindly read the entire manuscript: Cameron Poles; Stacey Guthrie; Drs. Olga Bazhenova, Barbara Wasik, and Ronald Bailey; and professors Stephen Porges, Nathan Fox, John Guthrie, and Kathryn Wentzel.

Malcolm L. Call, senior editor at the University of Georgia Press, has been a helpful, knowing, and enthusiastic guide. It has been a pleasure to work with Jennifer Comeau, whose expertise was invaluable throughout the production process, and Kelly Caudle, who lent her considerable editing skills to this project.

Excerpts from this book appeared in the article "You Are Different Now," published in the Summer 2000 special issue of *Feminist Studies* on women and health.